AUTISM AND STANDARD OF LIVING

AUTISM AND STANDARD OF LIVING

UNDERSTANDING THE ENVIRONMENTAL CRISIS

ZIVOTA NIKOLIC

Autism and Standard of Living
Zivota Nikolic

Published by Spines
ISBN 979-8-90002-255-0

CONTENTS

PART II

DEDICATION

This book is dedicated to my late friend Eli, who died in a house fire on December 24, 1987. It was set up by his autistic son and his sister by accident with a radio cassette player, by leaving the cassette player laying down on the couch in the playroom. His wife and sister-in-law were Christmas shopping. Eli was in the jacuzzi resting after a long day.

I was at my house in Simi Valley in my bed listening to the local news station. At one point, I just heard news that in Canoga Park there was a house fire and one man died. A few seconds after that, I received a phone call to inform me that Eli died in the house fire and that I needed to go because the wife was not home and the kids were at the neighbor's house. I got in my car and drove as fast as I could to be there before his wife arrived. The front of the 2nd floor was gone completely. The Fire Chief that was in charge explained to me what happened, how it happened, and the place where they found Eli's body.

Now we had to see how his wife was going to react when she saw all this and how we were going to protect her from getting near a breakdown. This was a moment in my life that I am never going to forget, and every time I talk about it, tears come from my eyes. Now the boy is 50 years old and trying to learn how to live by himself because his mother is sick and can't take care of him. I knew the boy when he was a little baby. At that time, I didn't know anything about autism, but now I know how he got autism.

Instead of celebrating Orthodox Christmas on January 7, at my house we were laying Eli to rest. This tragic situation pushed me all my life to think about autism problems and how they could be resolved. We just need to understand our standard of living, and we will be much healthier.

Eli's name is Ilija Barovic, born in Montenegro.
His wife's name is Anka.
Autistic son: Danis.
And daughter: Maja.

ACKNOWLEDGMENT

In the United States, I tried to inform the CDC, FDA, and many other government institutions and officials, including my senators. Nobody responded to any of my emails or telephone calls. I even received comments that I couldn't submit any scientific work because I don't have an academic name.

Educating new parents this way is my only option to save millions of kids from developing autism. There is no medicine to restart a mother's cell to begin developing the brain center again. If you cut half of a finger off, you are going to have that finger short all your life; it is never going to grow back. That is exactly the same with a baby's brain center for different functions.

ABOUT THE AUTHOR

I don't intend to brag, but I have studied autism from a slightly different perspective than that of classical medical research. I have looked at how today's perceived improvements in the standard of living compared to the past may be the root cause of the increase in the rates of autism.

The last 50 years or so of research in the field of autism have not been able to explain the root cause of the rise in the rate of autism in babies and young children. From one case in thousands in the 1960s, we are now at the point of one case in 36 and even less.

Why? Well, there are several answers to that. Let's explore the reasons.

Academic medical research has been completely unable to come up with an explanation of the cause of autism and how to prevent and heal it.

Over the last decade, I have been researching the relationship between the immune system, oxygen concentration levels in the air we breathe, the levels of amino acids, and their effect on humans and warm-blooded animals.

A first consideration is that few houses and apartments

50 years ago had central heating and air conditioning systems. Therefore, ventilation in homes and apartments relied on outside air entering through windows. This outside air is important for replacing indoor air, which can reduce oxygen levels and increase carbon dioxide levels, essentially due to the breathing of humans and pets.

The outside air is composed primarily of 78.08% nitrogen, 20.90% oxygen, and .04% carbon dioxide. Carbon dioxide, which is the least by volume of the three main elements but the most toxic, weighs the most at approximately 44g per mole, oxygen weighs approximately 32g per mole, and nitrogen weighs approximately 18g per mole.

Proper ventilation of a building with outside air keeps the levels of oxygen and carbon dioxide concentration optimal from the floor to the ceiling of every room in a building. Without proper ventilation, the carbon dioxide that humans and pets breathe out, which is heavier than oxygen, stays close to the floor and pushes oxygen up. As a result, it increases the levels of carbon dioxide we breathe in above safe levels and reduces the oxygen levels that our bodies need to breathe in to remain healthy.

Over the past 50 years, houses, apartments, and buildings that have new heating, ventilation, and air conditioning (HVAC) systems have been designed with energy and cost efficiency to heat and cool inside air by recirculating inside air and with minimum ventilation from the outside. Often, the only access to outside air comes from the exhaust of the tiny bathroom fan, only when it is turned on.

For proper ventilation in our homes, we need to have windows or sliding doors that extend all the way down to the floor, with an exhaust fan in one of them. Every other window should also have the ability to open the intake panel from the bottom of the floor. We can also use modern wireless technology to design windows and doors that can automatically and regularly open sufficiently for proper ventilation. Proper ventilation is similar to using a broom correctly to sweep the floor. We need to sweep that toxic air, carbon dioxide, ideally on a daily basis, in places where we and our pets spend time.

The same basic principle applies to hotel rooms that may be clean and well-maintained, but often lack fresh air unless they have windows that can be opened. Stale air is noticeable upon checking in, unless the windows were open during a recent room cleaning. Without windows, the only exhaust air exits through bathroom fans, and the new air comes under the room door from recirculated indoor air. This process equalizes atmospheric pressure but does not effectively equalize oxygen levels.

Oxygen concentration levels in our homes and places of work that fall below the 20.9% level found in the outside air are very bad for our health. Each percentage of oxygen concentration breathed in below 20.9% translates to 4.785% less oxygen in the bloodstream than our bodies need to be healthy.

Concentrated carbon dioxide is the deadliest gas on Earth. People who are subject to toxic levels of carbon dioxide exhibit no warning symptoms. They simply collapse and die.For example, in wineries, fermentation is performed in rooms that have window openings below the ceilings and above the floors. That is the safest way to ventilate the room, ensuring workers do not die from toxic concentrations of carbon dioxide generated from the fermentation process.

The oxygen concentration levels of some of the homes, apartments, office buildings, schools, hotels, and shopping malls that I measured showed as little as 17.9% oxygen concentration levels, 3% less than 20.9%, meaning that the people spending time there were getting 14.35% (3-4.785) less oxygen in their bloodstream compared to healthy levels.

Lower oxygen concentration reduces atmospheric pressure, resulting in energy savings required by city building ordinances, but it also increases the concentration of toxic air breathed in by humans. When we open an outside door to a building with a modern HVAC system, the air rushing in feels as though it has a higher oxygen concentration. This equalizes atmospheric pressure, but not oxygen concentration.

Unless all the air inside a building is continually replaced by outside air with ventilation, the oxygen concentration levels inside the building will not be the same as outside and will be below 20.9%. If we want to spend our days and nights in a healthy environment, especially our bedrooms, classrooms, and workplaces, we need to evaluate the standards by which the modern buildings we spend our time in have been designed for ventilation.

- To a natural standard, like living with no walls or in a tent? No.
- To a full ventilation system standard that exchanges inside air completely with outside air? No.
- To a standard of ventilation that eliminates the heaviest elements of air, such as toxins that negatively affect the quality of our health, such as carbon dioxide? Not at all.
- Is the bathroom fan strong enough to pull heavier air from the floor level and send it outside? Absolutely not.

Let's examine how this oxygen and carbon dioxide dynamic can affect babies and young children.

So, if we purchase a crib that has a typical minimum size of 28" by 52" with solid ends and sides that are lined with cushions, the crib effectively becomes a closed-in bucket with little to no circulation where the baby lies. This is an unhealthy sleeping space for a baby.

If this crib is placed in a room with an HVAC system or poor ventilation as described above, carbon dioxide from the room will settle into the crib. Additionally, the carbon dioxide generated by the baby's breathing while they sleep or play will also remain in the crib.

Even when the baby is taken out of the crib, without proper ventilation, the carbon dioxide in the crib will remain and be present when the baby is returned to the crib. It will continue to accumulate and increase in concentration each day if there is no adequate ventilation in the crib and room.

Furthermore, as the baby grows, so does their lung capacity, which increases the amount of carbon dioxide they exhale with each breath. Too much carbon dioxide in the bloodstream can create blood clots that may plug capillary blood vessels, preventing mother cells that are developing in certain brain centers from reproducing and transmitting. These cells eventually die and cannot reproduce in this situation, creating scars in the brain.

These blood clots and scars are what cause autism. The longer a baby stays in a crib with poor ventilation, the greater the probability that they may suffer blood clots and scars that result in brain damage, causing autism.

Each autistic child has different behavioral symptoms that are explained by the fact that the brain damage they have been subject to occurs in different parts of the brain and at different stages of development of the brain that affect the functions for social skills, speaking, hearing, coordination and controlling the movements, etc.

The changes and evolution of the concentration of carbon dioxide over a period of time in baby cribs can be mathematically proven. With the dimensions of the baby crib, the breath rate of the baby, and the lung capacity of the baby, we can determine the concentration of carbon dioxide generated from the baby's breath that remains in the crib, which can be confirmed with devices that measure carbon dioxide and oxygen concentration levels.

The pressure generated by a baby's breath is not strong enough to push carbon dioxide far away from their nose and mouth. In their next breath, they inhale part of the carbon dioxide that they have just breathed out, increasing the carbon dioxide concentration in their bloodstream that creates blood clots in capillary vessels and causes their brain center's mother cells to die, creating scars on those parts of the brain that will therefore not be able to transmit and develop.

Blood clots and scarring that occur at different brain development times are the reason that autistic children have differing symptoms. The fact that the large majority of children of the same age with autism are boys rather than girls is explained by the fact that the lungs of boys have greater capacity than those of girls of the same age and weight. As explained above, we can calculate the buildup of carbon dioxide concentrations for the time spent in a crib. Because their lung capacity is lower, girls have a lower probability of blood clotting, scarring, and brain damage.

Sudden infant death syndrome can also be explained by carbon dioxide toxicity. This analysis can be easily tested with laboratory rats and mice. If they are put in one bucket with no holes on the bottom, and a second bucket has holes drilled in the bottom, raise the buckets 12 inches from the floor and have the same number and same age animals with plentiful food and water, the one in the bucket with holes will be fine for a long time. But in the bucket with no holes, after some time, they will desperately try to climb out of the bucket and will soon get sick and die.

The solution to the autism problem is to ensure that baby cribs do not have solid pillow and blanket-laden sides and that the concentration levels of carbon dioxide in the rooms in which they spend their time do not exceed .04%. Proper ventilation in the rooms that babies spend their time in, including hospital rooms and special beds they may be placed in because of jaundice and other conditions, will ensure that oxygen levels do not fall below 20.9% and carbon dioxide levels do not rise above .04%.

The noses and mouths of babies need to be free of obstacles. Ideal cribs are playpens with bottoms that can be lowered as the baby grows and starts to stand until they can be moved into a bed. Along with a proper crib, proper ventilation of their room remains vital, especially in rooms in houses with HVAC systems and without windows and sliding doors that ventilate air at the level of the floor.

All doctors and medical practitioners involved in childbirth should be educated on this knowledge. They should transmit this information to expecting parents as part of the prenatal process. If this is done, it will take a matter of a couple of years before rates of autism go back to where they were more than 50 years ago, to one in every few hundred thousand of childbirths.

We can compare how parents cared for their babies 50 years ago to how parents care for their babies today. If we compare baby cribs from 50 years ago to the baby cribs sold in stores today, we will find that the cribs have changed.

Through my research, I have discovered that in addition to autism, obesity rates also started to increase when government building codes replaced swamp coolers with HVAC systems in the Southern states of the United States.

The Centers for Disease Control (CDC) has data relating to obesity on Indian reservations pre- and post-installation of HVAC systems on those reservations that substantiate this impact.

It can also be inferred that many other neurological challenges of children, adults, and senior citizens are caused or enhanced by excess carbon dioxide and lack of oxygen in bedrooms, schools, workspaces, hospitals, senior living spaces, and other buildings.

PREFACE

Over time, autism has become a significant issue for humanity, extending beyond any specific country or community. In this book, we will explore the dramatic increase in autism rates over the past few decades and examine the connection between modern living standards and this rise.

Additionally, we will discuss how poorly ventilated indoor environments, particularly those with high CO2 levels, may be a key, overlooked factor affecting early brain development. From the perspectives of science and architecture, this book will challenge conventional views that focus solely on genetics or vaccines. We will also reevaluate how we design and inhabit our living spaces to better protect children's neurological health, ultimately enhancing their overall quality of life.

PART I

CHAPTER 1

THE UNPRECEDENTED RISE OF AUTISM IN MODERN SOCIETY

The world is full of children, each with their own unique way of experiencing life. Some children, however, stand out—not because of what they do but because of how they see and interact with the world around them. Some rarely smile or struggle to find the words to express themselves. Some shy away from the chaos of social interactions, finding solace in solitude instead. While these behaviors can stem from countless causes, one possibility lingers in the shadows: autism.

Autism doesn't hide in the corners of society—it exists all around us, touching the lives of children in our families, schools, and communities. It could be your sibling, child, friend, or even a quiet colleague at work. If you're holding this book, chances are you've already crossed paths with someone on the autism spectrum—or perhaps you're navigating that journey right now. This is where understanding begins.

Before we dive deep and explore numbers, as well as

the reasons for the rise of autism cases in the world, it is important to understand what autism actually is.

Autism, which is also referred to as Autism Spectrum Disorder (ASD), is a developmental problem that impacts the way a human being interacts with the world around them.

The brain of a person suffering from autism cannot process sights, smells, and sounds the same way an average person's brain does. Moreover, people with autism also have a hard time expressing their emotions. Other than that, they struggle with speech, repetitive behaviors like picking skin and neck movements, as well as anger problems.

Usually, autism is diagnosed at an early age, and the symptoms may vary from one person to another. Sometimes, they may not respond to their own name, even if it is in their mother's tone of voice. Moreover, they have a hard time making eye contact and engaging in social activities, and they mostly prefer staying alone.

One may also find them too preoccupied with a specific object and may also be disturbed, provided there is a change in their daily routine. Such children also lack the smile one would expect from a normal child. Also, they are sensitive to bright lights, noise, and loud colors.

With time, considerable research has been carried out on the topic of autism, and several treatments have been discovered. Some of the most common treatments for autism include applied behavior therapy, physical and occupational therapy, picture exchange communication systems, and sensory integration therapy. Then there are medications, which aren't necessarily aimed at curing autism, but they help with issues like impulsiveness, seizures, insomnia, and depressive episodes.

Autism Rates Around the World

In the U.S., one in 36 children suffers from some kind of autism. Numbers show that over 67 million people worldwide are affected by autism. If we look at numbers from the U.S., boys are four times more likely to experience autism than their female counterparts. According to a 2020 figure by the Centers for Disease Control, one in 59 children has been diagnosed with autism. While it is a sad reality, the fact of the matter is that the number of autism cases in the U.S. is slightly higher than the global average.[1]

In the UK, the number drops to one in 100, which is similar to the figures in Australia. According to the National Autistic Society, approximately 700,000 people in the UK are found on the autism spectrum, and over half of those people are children.[2]

In Canada, the estimates suggest that one in 66 individuals is on the autism spectrum, and the prevalence is similar to that in the U.S. According to the Indian Journal of Psychiatry, the number in India is one in 250 people,

---

1. Autism Statistics & Facts: How many people have autism? (n.d.). https://www.thetreetop.com/statistics/autism-prevalence
2. National Autistic Society & National Autistic Society. (n.d.). What is Autism? https://www.autism.org.uk/advice-and-guidance/what-is-autism#:~:text=Autism%20is%20a%20lifelong%20developmental,and%20children%20in%20the%20UK.

which is also the number seen in Brazil. In China, the number drops to one in 186 people, which is lower than the figures in the U.S., UK, Brazil, India, and Australia. In South Africa, one out of 160 people is on the spectrum of autism.

Autism Rates Since the 1960s

In the 1960s and 70s, 2-4 children out of a total of 10,000 were diagnosed with autism. Today, the number is 100 times higher. In the U.S., the numbers have risen by 1000% from 1 in 500 in the 1970s to 1 in 36 today.

In the UK, the figures have gone up by 500%, from one in 1000 in 1990 to one in 100. In Canada, autism cases have gone up by 500%, from one in 2000 to one in 66. In Australia, the figures have increased by 400%, from one in 2500 to one in 100.

Since 2002, the autism numbers in India have shot up by 400%. In 2002, one in 2000 people would be diagnosed with autism.

Today, it is one in 250 in India. In China, there has been a 600% increase in autism cases. In 2000, the number was one in 1667, and today, that number stands at a staggering one in 186.

In Brazil, the numbers have gone up by 500% since the year 2000. From one in 2000, the figure has gone up to one in 250. Shockingly, South Africa has reported a considerable rise in autism cases. Since the year 2000, autism numbers have increased by 700%. From one in 1429 to 2000, the number now stands at one in 160.

Reasons for the Rise in Autism Cases

When it comes to evaluating the root causes of autism, there is no one-size-fits-all approach. Different people can have different reasons triggering their condition. However, let's break down the different reasons that may result in Autism Spectrum Disorder, and they may vary from one person to another.

Better Diagnosis and Increased Awareness

With time, the definition of Autism has actually expanded. Now, pervasive developmental disorders and disorders like Asperger's Syndrome also fall within the umbrella of ASD. Moreover, medical practitioners now have better access to the latest resources and screening tools that allow them to diagnose the issue earlier on.

The best part is that public awareness has also increased during the past few decades, and people are more and more mindful of their health, as well as their children's health, especially mental, psychological, and emotional health. What's even more promising is that the diagnosis of Autism has become easier and quicker in underprivileged minority groups, which is why we see more cases today than two decades ago.

Hereditary and Genetic Influence

According to research, if one child in the family has autism, chances are that the ones that will come later might also experience the same. Similarly, spontaneous gene mutations in the early stages of fetal development can also result in children having ASD. Parental age also plays a key role. According to research, children who are born to older parents, and especially fathers over the age of 40, are likely to develop autism.[3]

Prenatal and Environmental Factors

One of the causes of autism in children is prenatal exposure, which includes air pollution exposure and exposure to toxic chemicals during pregnancy. Then comes maternal health. Various conditions, including high blood pressure, diabetes, and obesity during pregnancy, can result in autism. The medications the mother takes during pregnancy can also lead to ASD. According to research, some medications, such as valproic acid, which is used to control epilepsy, can result in autism in the offspring. Similarly, babies that are born prematurely or are born with low body weight are likely to experience ASD.[4]

---

3. Jewel Centre For Autism. (2025, January 28). Why Are Autism Rates Rising? Causes & Facts Explained. Jewel Autism Centre and Child Development Centre. https://www.jewelautismcentre.com/the-rising-autism-rates-what-factors-are-contributing-to-this-increase/
4. MGH Center for Women's Mental Health. (2015, August 6). Exposure to valproic acid and increased risk of autism spectrum disorders - MGH Center for Women's Mental Health. MGH Center for Women's Mental Health - Perinatal & Reproductive Psychiatry at Mass General Hospital.

Societal and Lifestyle Changes

Modern parents are more interested in researching independently and seeking professional help, if needed. Hence, they are aware of developmental milestones, as well as the help they may need with their children. As a result, autism is diagnosed earlier in life, which results in higher numbers. Another reason is the changes in early lifestyle. Increased screen time, less green time, lack of social interactions, and poor eating habits are some of the potential reasons that may lead to autism in children.

The Modern Environment and Rise in Autism Spectrum Disorder

The prevalence of ASD has considerably increased, especially in recent decades, moving from 1 in 150 children in 2000 to 1 in 54 children in 2020 in the United States. Such a rapid rise suggests that environmental factors play a key role. While the human genome has remained relatively stable all these years, modern life comes up with numerous potential triggers, which include xenobiotics, immune system dysregulation, as well as the constant stress of a rapidly changing environment.

One of the key factors is immune system dysregulation. Modern diets, gut dysbiosis, and exposure to xenobiotics can result in an immune system imbalance, which affects brain development. According to research, maternal

---

https://womensmentalhealth.org/posts/exposure-to-valproic-acid- and-increased-risk-of-autism-spectrum-disorders/

immune activation during pregnancy can increase autism risk. Furthermore, 70-75% of children with ASD exhibit an immune system that impacts folate receptors on brain cells, which further hinders crucial functions like DNA repair and neurotransmitter production. The FRAT test helps identify these antibodies, while treatments, such as leucovorin, have shown promising results.[5]

Another contributor that cannot be undermined is the proliferation of xenobiotics, which are chemical substances foreign to the biological systems of the human body. Furthermore, pesticides, industrial chemicals, and other pollutants can play a key role in disrupting neurological development.

Studies have correlated prenatal exposure to certain pesticides with the increased risk of autism. Reducing exposure to pesticides, properly filtering drinking water, and eating organic foods are some of the recommended techniques to mitigate these effects. Moreover, infectious diseases and the changing landscape of microbial exposure may also play their part, with maternal infections during pregnancy linked to higher autism rates.[6]

The rampant changes and high levels of environmental stimuli in modern life can also influence gene expression

---

5. Shelton, J. F., et al. (2014). Neurodevelopmental Disorders and Prenatal Residential Proximity to Agricultural Pesticides: The CHARGE Study. Environmental Health Perspectives, 122(10), 1103-1109.

6. Román, P., Ruiz-González, C., Rueda-Ruzafa, L., Cardona, D., Requena, M., & Alarcón, R. (2024). Exposure to environmental pesticides and the risk of autism spectrum Disorders: a Population-Based Case-Control study. Medicina, 60(3), 479. https://doi.org/10.3390/medicina60030479

through epigenetic mechanisms. The stress of modern living can result in neuroinflammation, which is linked to neurodevelopmental disorders such as autism.

Modifying the environment to minimize harmful exposures, improve diet, and minimize stress can positively impact individuals with ASD. While autism likely existed in the past, the current rise in cases appears to be driven by the interaction between genetic predisposition and these modern environmental factors, which aren't always the healthiest.

Sealed Living Spaces and Lack of Ventilation

Gone are the days when people lived in open areas with ample greenery and fresh air to benefit from. As urbanization grew, sealed living spaces became the norm. While they were safer than their open counterparts, they failed to offer the right amount of ventilation, which is instrumental in creating a safe living space.

Chances are, you spend a good amount of time and energy mopping that beautiful marble floor or the gorgeous rug in your living room. Does it mean you are not exposed to indoor contaminants and pollutants? Think again.

The indoor space may appear safe to the naked eye, but it is home to a myriad of pollutants like Volatile organic compounds (VOCs), pesticides, radon, cigarette smoke, asbestos, CO2, nitrogen dioxide, pet dander, dust, lead, moisture, mold, mildew, pollen, formaldehyde, particulate matter, and viruses that make us sick.

As much as you try to avoid it, and as you read this

very chapter, you are being exposed to all those pollutants. Now, think for a minute about being pregnant or raising a small child in such a sealed and suffocated environment. The chances of your children developing autism still exist until you allow them to venture out and let the fresh breeze fill up their lungs while filtering out the unhealthy elements that pollute their system.

People are often curious why countries like Kenya, with limited resources, have fewer cases of autism. While the social stigma and lack of resources and awareness cannot be denied, those countries have sufficient open spaces where people and their children can breathe freely without being exposed to the most dangerous of pollutants.

Final Word

With time, the approach to life, which once was totally hands-on, has been replaced with a more digital approach. As a result, people do not use their bodies for the purpose they are intended for.

As a result, they are becoming lazier, more lethargic, and mentally weaker compared to the people who came before them. For a human being and their offspring to experience healthy neurological development, they need to have the full 360-degree human experience, which comes from moving their bodies, sweating, making the blood flow in their veins, and burning energy to create new energy, even if it requires them to get their hands dirty in the process.

During this ordeal, they are most likely to experience the gifts of Mother Nature, like sunlight, wind, water, and the smell of soil. If we can prioritize all of these things, the chances of autism and similar neurological problems can be avoided.

CHAPTER 2

REDEFINING OUR UNDERSTANDING OF AUTISM DEVELOPMENT

If you currently know someone with autism or have at some point in life, it is crucial to understand the connection between ASD and brain development. Usually, the earliest changes to the brain take place during the first two years of life, which is usually before the child is diagnosed with autism.

According to research, children who are diagnosed later show signs of faster autism growth in specific areas of the brain. For example, children with ASD tend to showcase faster cortex surface expansion. This expansion rate is six to 12 months faster than their non-autistic counterparts. The early growth of autism is more significant, and it often tends to correlate with the signs that may show up later on.[1]

In autistic children, changes to brain surface area and volume are significant. As traits of autism become more

---

1. Autism and brain development interconnection. (n.d.). https://www.mastermindbehavior.com/post/autism-and-the-brain-development#

apparent in older siblings, their younger siblings may also experience alterations in brain volume and surface area.

When talking about the impacts of autism on brain development and growth, the genetic factors cannot be forgotten. Certain hereditary influences have a key impact on how the brain grows and its networks connect. Some people who lack the corpus callosum or some part of it are more likely to experience signs of autism. The corpus callosum is the part that connects the two hemispheres of the brain. This observation shows that disruption in neural connections can lead to autistic symptoms.

Structural Variances

When understanding how autism affects brain development, it is important for us to understand the structural variances. Some of the key areas include cortical growth, cerebellum, and hippocampus.

Cortical Growth

According to studies, the surface area of the cortex increases between ages six and 12 months. During the second year of their lives, autistic children tend to showcase faster increases in brain volume, which is different from non-autistic children.[2]

---

2. Askham, A. V. (2024, October 1). Brain structure changes in autism, explained. The Transmitter: Neuroscience News and Perspectives. https://www.thetransmitter.org/spectrum/brain-structure-changes- in-autism-explained/

This cortical growth can affect a child's social and cognitive skills, which highlights the complexity of brain development in autistic children.

Cerebellum Abnormalities

The cerebellum exists at the base of the human skull. This part is also helpful in understanding the brain development of autistic individuals. Autistic children tend to have extra tissue in different parts of the cerebellum. While the cerebellum is usually associated with motor coordination, its role has expanded to social interactions and cognitive functions as well. These abnormalities in the cerebellum result not only in physical problems but also in emotional problems.[3]

Hippocampus Enlargement

Children with autism showcase an enlarged hippocampus. This part of the brain is responsible for memory and storage. The enlargement of the hippocampus is common among autistic children, but it is unclear whether this enlargement follows them into adulthood. Another common observation is the one related to the amygdala, which is used for processing emotions. This part can be bigger or smaller in children with autism. This

---

3. Askham, A. V. (2024b, October 1). Brain structure changes in autism, explained. The Transmitter: Neuroscience News and Perspectives. https://www.thetransmitter.org/spectrum/brain-structure-changes- in-autism-explained/

inconsistency in the size of the amygdala calls for further research.

Neuroanatomical Aspects

In this section, we will look at three key aspects: neuronal connectivity, amygdala size differences, and neocortex alterations.

Amygdala Size

According to research, toddlers with ASD tend to experience increases in the size of the right and left sides of their amygdala, which is different from children who are neurotypical. Such an enlargement has a positive correlation with communication and social interaction issues. It is also important to understand that the volume changes in the amygdala depend on age. While the growth may be faster during childhood, it can slow down as the child grows up. According to research, the size of the amygdala can result in emotional problems in boys and girls suffering from autism, especially girls.[4]

Alterations in the Neocortex

This part of the brain is responsible for some higher-level functions. Alterations in the neocortex are commonly

4. Autism and brain development interconnection. (n.d.-b). https://www.mastermindbehavior.com/post/autism-and-the-brain-development#

noticed in children with autism. According to some studies, brain tissue samples from autistic children tend to identify 194 genes, which are different from those of neurotypical brains. Furthermore, such alterations tend to include an upregulation of over 140 genes that produce more mRNA, whereas a downregulation of genes that produce 51 genes that produce less mRNA. The ones that are downregulated are the ones related to brain connectivity. This may have an impact on the efficiency of neuronal communication.

Neuronal Connectivity

Neuronal connectivity refers to how the neurons communicate while forming networks within the brain. According to research, the connectivity patterns within the brain can be disrupted by autism. This disruption can change the way a person processes and responds to information. The downregulation of neocortex genes highlights issues in neuron communication, as well as the overall connectivity of the brain.

Factors Influencing the Development of the Brain

When it comes to understanding the impacts of autism on the human brain, it is vital to understand the genetic and environmental factors. Not only does it help us understand how these factors not only shape the development of autism, but also determine how it manifests itself.

Genetic Factors

According to research, genetic factors contribute to 40-80% of the risk of developing autism. In similar research, changes to over 1000 genes have been linked to ASD. In 2% to 4% of people suffering from autism, genetic mutations are said to be the underlying cause. Such mutations often affect singular genes that are responsible for brain development and thus influence synaptic function, dendrite development, organization, growth, and neuron production.

Similarly, the father's age and the mother's health condition during pregnancy may also play a key role in the child developing autistic symptoms. If the father is over 34 years of age, or if the mother has suffered from metabolic syndrome, infections during pregnancy, or mental health problems like depression, anxiety, or severe stress, these conditions can contribute to autism in children.

Environmental Factors

Environmental factors work closely with genetic factors, thus affecting the development of the brain. Just like the mother's health, prenatal medications also lead to autism. Painkillers and antiepileptic medicines have also been linked to higher rates of autism. Similarly, other environmental factors like air quality, pollutants, and ventilation play a significant role in the development of ASD at an early age.

These factors tend to disrupt normal neurodevelopment. This highlights the relationship between the environment and genetics in shaping the characteristics of autism, as well as its impact on the brain. Only by understanding the genetic and environmental factors can we better comprehend how autism affects the development of the brain.

Air Quality, Pollution, and Brain Development

When we talk about the causes of autism, most research is aimed at the genetic causes, which is fine. However, environmental factors are just as important, especially the ones related to air quality and pollution.

In 2020, some researchers at the University of California found a direct correlation between air pollution and the increase in risk to brain development, which can further result in neurodevelopmental disorders. Their study was based on rodent models, the previous studies that showed such an association.[5]

Sure, air pollution has been a known cause of cardiovascular problems. However, during the last five to 10 years, scientists have taken a keen interest in its impact on the human brain. Previously, the researchers had worked on the effects of proximity to busy roadways on brain development. However, the data on traffic-related air pollution and its impact on the brain were almost non-existent.

---

5. Air quality impacts early brain development. (2020, December 5). School of Veterinary Medicine. https://www.vetmed.ucdavis.edu/news/air-quality-impacts-early- brain-development

Understanding this void of unavailable information, UC Davis toxicologist Pamela Lein stepped in. Lein worked closely with atmospheric scientist Anthony Wexler and Kelly Petten, a doctoral student of toxicology and pharmacology. Lein wanted to come up with a novel approach to studying the impacts of traffic-related pollution in a real-time fashion.

The three scientists ended up setting up a vivarium close to a busy traffic tunnel in California. To mimic the human experience as closely as possible, they used a rodent as a test subject. According to Lein, it is important for people to understand if it is risky to live close enough to a busy roadway, and if it is, it would be easier for doctors and scientists to warn pregnant females, or parents whose children have already been diagnosed with a neurodevelopmental problem, so they may seek help, and take the right steps to prevent further damage.

In this study, the scientists compared the brains of two different groups of rat pups. One group was exposed to clean air, while the other was exposed to polluted air. By the time the results came out, scientists had seen that the brains of rat pups exposed to polluted air were suffering from severe neuroinflammation.

It shows that exposure to pollution, especially during the formative years, can affect brain development. According to Petten, the changes noticed during this study are subtle. However, these effects were seen in air pollution that falls within the limits of regulation.

For children to experience neurodevelopmental issues in their early years, they may have to go through the cumulative effect of genetic and environmental factors. Petten also said that in the environment, we can find certain particulate matter that is not yet regulated, but it still exists, wreaking havoc on the brains of our young ones, who are still in their formative years.

Final Word

The medical community's current approach to research on ASD is significantly shaped by pharmaceutical funds and the money that comes from established academic groups, which often prioritize drug treatments and biological factors. Pharmaceutical companies fund much of the research, focusing on medications, such as SSRIs, to manage symptoms like anxiety, which can limit attention to non-pharmacological approaches like behavioral therapies.

As far as academic frameworks are concerned, they typically treat autism as a neurological disorder that needs to be fixed, thus aligning with pharmaceutical interests and often overlooking social, cultural, and, most importantly, environmental influences.

Critics on this issue often argue that this narrow focus results in a rather reductionist view of autism, thus ignoring its complexity, as well as the diverse experiences of individuals on the spectrum. Furthermore, pharmaceutical funding can create a form of bias, which can potentially distort research outcomes. A more inclusive approach is needed to address these limitations, incorporating environmental, social, and psychological factors.

The neurodiversity movement emphasizes acceptance

of autism as a natural variation and advocates for a broader definition of success, focusing on improving the quality of life of autistic individuals and inclusion rather than just symptom reduction.

While pharmaceutical and biological research is important, a more comprehensive and balanced approach that considers various factors and the lived experiences of individuals with autism is essential for advancing autism research and improving outcomes for those affected.

CHAPTER 3

THE SILENT THREAT: UNDERSTANDING CO2 IN INDOOR ENVIRONMENTS

Remember science class in grade school? In those lectures, one of the frequently discussed gases was carbon dioxide. But what is carbon dioxide? Simply put, carbon dioxide is carbon's naturally occurring oxide, which is found in trace quantities. As much as we are wary of the harmful effects of CO2 on human health, there is no running away from it, as it exists everywhere in varying quantities.

This gas is formed when the central atom, carbon, covalently bonds with two atoms of oxygen through double bonds. CO2 can be synthetically produced by various industrial processes. Whether it is the food and beverage industry, life jackets, or fire extinguishers, all contribute to the creation of CO2. This greenhouse gas is also a key component of the process of photosynthesis. Despite its adverse health impacts, carbon dioxide is important for several applications on a day-to-day basis.

Before we move forward and talk about CO2 in our indoor spaces, it is important to understand the physical properties of this gas. CO2 tends to exist naturally in the gaseous form with a molar mass of 44 $g{\cdot}mol^{-1}$ and a melting point of -55.6°C. Below this temperature, carbon dioxide can be found in a solid state.

This solid form of CO2 is known as dry ice. It is important to understand that it shouldn't come into contact with bare skin, as it can result in skin damage. Being a covalent and linear molecule, CO2 is slightly soluble in water. However, with an increase in temperature, its water solubility is likely to decrease.

In the gaseous state, CO2 lacks color and odor. However, it is slightly sour in taste. CO2 is a dense gas, with a density of 1.977gmL-1. As a result, it is heavier than air and can displace oxygen. Furthermore, it possesses an acidic nature and, when mixed with water, can create an acid known as carbonic acid. The acid is weak and can turn a blue litmus paper red.

The good news is that carbon dioxide is not flammable, which is why it is used in fire extinguishers. Remember, the process of combustion requires oxygen. What CO2 does is it cuts the oxygen supply from the fuel source. The combustion reaction of CO2 is as follows.

$$O2 + Ch4 \rightarrow Co2 + H2O$$

When found in higher concentrations, CO2 tends to have a pungent odor and can prove toxic to human health. In the event that a person is exposed to pure and unfiltered CO2 without the slightest supply of oxygen, they may collapse and die. However, if the concentration remains low, CO2 isn't as toxic and remains odorless.

Day-to-Day Activities Leading to CO2 Accumulation

For a while now, the conversations surrounding climate change have become a staple in academic and healthcare circles. As a result, a fair chunk of the population is now interested in talking about the CO2 accumulation within their home. Before we move toward the specifics, it is important to understand that CO2 buildup can lead to concentration loss, dizziness, fatigue, headaches, and shortness of breath.

As we have discussed above, CO2 is all around us, and if its concentration goes beyond 1000 PPM, it can affect a person's health and well-being.[1]

However, awareness of the sources of CO2 accumulation in your homes can help you keep it to a safer level. Similarly, architects can also take the necessary steps to address climate change while minimizing the future impacts of CO2.[2]

Daniel Jaconetti serves as the national sustainable design leader at HED. According to Jaconetti, the best

---

1. Prill, R. (n.d.). Why measure carbon dioxide inside buildings? In Washington State University Extension Energy Program. https://www.energy.wsu.edu/documents/co2inbuildings.pdf
2. Rote, L. (2025, February 14). How architects can design for climate change. Gb&D Magazine. https://gbdmagazine.com/design-for-climate-change/

houses are the ones that are resilient, comfortable, energy-efficient, and don't contain toxic chemicals.

That said, let's look at some of the most common sources of CO2 accumulation within modern indoor living spaces.

HVAC Systems

The purpose of an HVAC system is to control the atmosphere. However, in the absence of proper ventilation, CO2 buildup can take place. A CO2 sensor can come in handy. It is important for the HVAC system to have a CO2 sensor. We can also maintain the effectiveness of our HVAC system by using filters and changing them in a timely fashion. Filters help reduce the amount of dust and debris in the air ducts.

Fireplace

The process of combustion can result in the production of several gases, and CO2 is one of them. In the absence of proper ventilation, fireplaces can indeed cause the buildup of toxic gases. CO2 monitors and smoke detectors can help solve this problem. Periodic professional inspections can also help mitigate the risk.

Laundry Rooms

According to research published in the Journal of Integrative Environmental Sciences, laundry rooms tend to emit at least 179 million metric tons of carbon dioxide per annum.[3] Most of this comes from dampness. High-spin cycles should be used before putting clothes into the dryer to minimize dampness. The less dampness there is, the quicker it will be for the clothes to dry. As a result, there will be fewer CO2 emissions. You can also reduce CO2 emissions by reducing the weekly load by washing only the clothes that are dirty.

Crowded Indoor Areas

According to studies, carbon dioxide makes up approximately 4% of the exhaled air. As a result, CO2 levels inside the living space tend to rise. If you have ever felt cramped or suffocated at a house party, you can credit a portion of that to the CO2 that exists within. You can start by opening windows for better air circulation and limiting the number of people within your indoor living space.[4]

Soil Underneath the Home

Interestingly, CO2 can remain trapped in the soil for several hundred years. As a result, the homes that are built

---

3. Golden, J. S., Subramanian, V., Irizarri, G. M. a. U., White, P., & Meier, F. (2010). Energy and carbon impact from residential laundry in the United Field Cod States. Journal of Integrative Environmental Sciences, 7(1), 53–73. https://doi.org/10.1080/19438150903541873.
4. Vranak, E. (2021, July 7). How to improve ventilation in a Post-Covid world. Gb&D Magazine. https://gbdmagazine.com/how-to-improve-ventilation/

on farms and landfills are more likely to have higher exposure to carbon due to their exposure to the organisms that live in the soil. However, by practicing no-till gardening and leaving the ground undisturbed, carbon can be kept in its place without being let out into the air we breathe.

Cigarette Smoking

Smoking is linked to several health problems, like cardiovascular issues and cancer. Moreover, smoking can also result in the accumulation of CO2. It is important to understand that the CO2 produced by cigarettes is 200 times more than that present in the atmosphere. Smoking inside can increase exposure to CO2 in a very major way.[5]

Stovetops

There is a reason why gas stoves come with range hoods. These hoods aren't merely for show. Instead, they exist to keep smoke, heat, grease, and moisture at bay. One must make sure to use the range hood when cooking to prevent CO2 accumulation. You can also open one of the windows or turn on the exhaust fan when cooking on a gas stove.

---

5. Schwartz, L., Guais, A., Chaumet-Riffaud, P., Grévillot, G., Sasco, A. J., Molina, T. J., & Abolhassani, M. (2010). Carbon dioxide is largely responsible for the acute inflammatory effects of tobacco smoke. Inhalation Toxicology, 22(7), 543–551. https://doi.org/10.3109/08958370903555909

Outdated Electrical Systems

The '70s were the first time in history when energy conservation became a focus in homes. At the time, using less energy was prime advice for people to conserve resources. If you live in a home that was built years and years ago, the best you can do is to replace the old heating and cooling systems with electrical ones to minimize CO2 within your living spaces.

Modern Homes and the Myth of Good Indoor Air Quality

One of the most common misconceptions is that newly built homes cannot have bad indoor air quality. In fact, the reality is quite the opposite of what most people believe. There are a variety of reasons why the air inside newly built homes can be far worse than the air inside older ones.

To begin with, it is the construction materials, new furniture, carpets, and linens that are still outgassing, i.e., releasing chemical fumes, and this process continues for several weeks and even months. Moreover, the dust from the entire construction process has yet to be removed. As a result, the super fine particulate matter may remain suspended within your home. Similarly, the unpacking and unboxing process can release contaminants into the air.

Houses today are built more tightly than before, keeping energy efficiency in mind. However, these modern designs have a tradeoff hidden somewhere. With modern houses, the tradeoff is the lack of fresh air entering your living space, in exchange for the reduced energy bill you pay at the end of the month. As a result, you end up with higher CO_2 levels in your living space.

Furthermore, a synergistic relationship exists between CO_2 levels and Volatile Organic Chemicals. Increased CO_2 levels allude to poor ventilation, not only for human occupants, but also for the proper outgassing of the chemical fumes we have discussed earlier. This is the reason why CO_2 levels above 1000 PPM can result in sick building syndrome (SBS).

In addition, the chemoreceptors located in the human body are found in the carotid arteries, aorta, and the brain. They tend to respond to increased CO_2 levels, which results in an increased breathing rate. When the breathing rate increases, dust tends to enter the lungs, as well as the bloodstream.

Overt exposure to CO_2 can result in CO_2 toxicity. Some of the most common symptoms include shortness of breath, muscle tremors, sweaty skin, increased heart rate, dimmed sight, minimized hearing, dizziness, drowsiness, confusion, headache, high blood pressure, and mild narcosis.

Increasing CO_2 concentrations have significant impacts on both indoor and outdoor environments. To address this, buildings have become more energy-efficient, often by improving airtightness. However, this can lead to poor air quality if proper ventilation is not maintained. In particular, airtight rooms can accumulate higher CO_2 levels, which could negatively affect occupant health and comfort.

Impact of CO2 Build-Up on Developing Brains

High CO2 concentrations can seriously impair cognitive abilities by minimizing the oxygen available to the human brain, especially in the early years. This happens due to the Bohr Effect, which was presented by Christian Bohr in 1904.[6]

In a 2016 study by Harvard University, cognitive performance significantly decreases as CO2 levels rise within indoor environments, especially between 900 and 1,400 ppm. The list of affected cognitive functions includes focus, strategic thinking, and information handling. The effect is more visible in children, and especially in exam settings, poor ventilation could result in CO2 levels exceeding 2,000 ppm, which severely impairs the child's performance.[7]

The guidelines recommend maintaining a daily average CO2 concentration of less than 1000 PPM. This is in line with the standards set by European countries such as Finland, Norway, and Germany. To achieve this, UK classrooms may need to exchange air within the room somewhere around five times an hour. This high air turnover is important to ensure the CO2 levels do not exceed the recommended threshold, thus maintaining a healthy learning environment for children.

---

6. Physiology, Bohr effect. (2025, January 1). PubMed. https://pubmed.ncbi.nlm.nih.gov/30252284/
7. The Headteacher | Better leadership, smarter spending. (n.d.). The Headteacher. https://www.theheadteacher.com/new-for-schools/the-impact-of-co2-on-childrens-learning

Poor air quality is a significant environmental threat, responsible for claiming 4.2 million lives in the UK alone. Children are particularly vulnerable to the long-term effects of pollution due to their still-developing lungs. Given these risks, it is crucial to prioritize better air quality in environments such as schools, where young individuals spend a considerable portion of their time.

One effective solution to reduce CO2 buildup and improve air quality is Mechanical Ventilation with Heat Recovery (MVHR). MVHR systems can recover nearly 90% of energy in a room by using an air-to-air heat exchanger to warm incoming air, thereby reducing heating demands and carbon footprints. This system provides fresh, filtered air, ensuring a well-ventilated space with lower pollution levels.

To enhance indoor air quality, classrooms must have fresh, filtered air with CO2 concentrations well under 1,000 ppm. Schools and institutions should actively assess and improve air quality to support the health and performance of their occupants, particularly in learning environments

Final Word

Carbon dioxide plays a key role in our everyday lives and the environment. However, its accumulation—especially in indoor spaces—can negatively impact human health and cognitive function, particularly in younger children. While CO2 is essential for various applications, from photosynthesis to fire extinguishers, excessive levels in closed environments can lead to discomfort and toxicity.

Modern homes present unique challenges. Tightly packed construction and lack of ventilation contribute to higher CO2 concentrations, which can impair cognitive performance in children. Given the evidence linking high CO2 levels to reduced cognitive function and health risks, it is vital to prioritize proper ventilation and adopt solutions like MVHR to ensure a healthy indoor environment.

As we build more energy-efficient homes, maintaining a balance between energy conservation and indoor air quality should be our utmost priority to protect human health and the environment.

CHAPTER 4

THE EVOLUTION OF LIVING SPACES: FROM NATURAL TO ARTIFICIAL ENVIRONMENTS

Over time, living spaces have truly evolved. That's right—smart homes are now the norm, and why shouldn't they be? Unlike the homes of the past, these homes tend to offer comfort, security, convenience, and energy efficiency. These houses are equipped to support heating, lighting, television systems, cameras, video games, and computers.

One of the things often brought up by the proponents of smart homes is how these homes have the power to conserve the Earth's natural resources. With built-in HVAC systems that have the ability to keep indoor air clean and safe for breathing, smart homes are really the answer to all the problems the human race has been facing since the dawn of time, or so it seems.

That said, smart homes aren't a recent invention. Instead, they have evolved into the smart and efficient homes that we see today.

It all started with the Industrial Revolution, around the year 1900, which spawned an entire race of machines in the form of electrical appliances to make life easier for humans.

As a result, we saw a barrage of machines that appeared in the form of dishwashers, washing machines, refrigerators, and vacuum cleaners. In the year 1930, scientists started thinking about automation. However, the idea didn't fully reach fruition until the 1960s when the first automation system dawned over the world. Then, in 1969, we saw the first kitchen computer.

Not only could it come up with creative recipes, but its affordability brought ample commercial success for the manufacturers. In the 1970s, we witnessed the emergence of microcontrollers, followed by the introduction of gerontechnology in the 1990s. By the early 2000s, the concept of smart homes began to take shape. Over time, home networking, home automation, domestic technologies, and various gadgets have been integrated into our living spaces. Now, with just a single click, everything can be controlled.

While smart homes may seem like the perfect solution for the problems faced by humans, they really aren't. Unlike the homes of the past, these smart homes have an HVAC system, which may seem helpful, but in reality, there are several gray areas. The good thing about the homes of the past was their natural ventilation, thus eliminating the dirt, mold, mildew, grime, pet dander, and cigarette smoke filling up our living spaces. As a result, it was easier to keep several allergies and respiratory and cardiovascular issues at bay.

This is one area where smart homes fail badly.

Furthermore, the buildup of pollutants inside the living space and the lack of natural ventilation profoundly impact the brain development of little children who are in their formative years. This stunted brain growth can result in neurological issues down the line and can also pave the way for Autism.

Modern Homes: Natural Ventilation vs. Artificial Ventilation

Back in the day, most homes had natural ventilation. However, with time, this natural ventilation was replaced by more mechanical ventilation and HVAC systems. However, with time, people have realized the effectiveness of natural ventilation, and they are turning back to it, thanks to the energy efficiency and eco-friendliness of natural ventilation. When compared to modern HVAC systems, natural ventilation can offer 10-30% more energy savings.

How Does It Work?

Simply put, natural ventilation is an approach that helps cool and ventilate buildings that receive a natural flow of air. With natural ventilation, exhaust fans and air-conditioners are rarely needed. In the process of doing its job, natural ventilation uses pressure and temperature differentials between the interior and exterior of the buildings for the purpose of facilitating air circulation, getting rid of stale, warm air, and allowing newer and cooler air to enter.

There are several variables on which the efficiency of a natural ventilation system is based. These variables include the placement and size of the openings, the prevalent patterns of wind, as well as the speed of air, and the temperature contrast that exists on the inside and the outside of the building.

When it comes to maximizing the effectiveness of natural ventilation systems, it is very important for us to factor in the architectural design, as well as the strategic placement of the openings.

The Benefits of Natural Ventilation

There are several benefits of natural ventilation.

- To begin with, it is a cost-effective form of climate control. It creates a comfortable indoor environment, especially on hot days. On days with higher temperatures, lack of ventilation can result in suffocation and excessive sweating, and it can also impact occupancy rates.
- One of the downsides of poor ventilation is poor health and lack of productivity among the occupants of a building. By creating an effectively ventilated building, we can create a workspace that is healthy and conducive to work.
- By incorporating natural ventilation in your building, you can align with the prescribed

safety standards, making indoor spaces safer and more user-friendly.

- Savings cannot be forgotten. The great thing about a natural ventilation system is how it uses the airflow on the outside to maintain the indoor climate, keeping it cool and minimizing your reliance on mechanical cooling systems. As a result, you can save enough money on energy costs.

Does Natural Ventilation Minimize Energy Costs?

The answer is yes. It does reduce energy costs. Here is how it does that:

- With natural ventilation, you don't need electricity 24/7. As a result, your energy costs go down considerably.
- Secondly, your maintenance expenses remain streamlined. Natural ventilation systems are simple. They lack many complex components. As a result, there is too little to maintain, which helps you save money considerably.
- Lastly, in several situations, natural ventilation helps you minimize your dependence on air-conditioning. In many cases, natural air eliminates the need for artificial air-conditioning, which consumes considerable energy. Not only does this slash away energy costs, but it also makes your efforts more energy-efficient and eco-friendly.

Building Standards Affecting Air Quality

We may not realize it, but it is a fact that buildings tend to contribute around 39% of global energy-related carbon emissions. Of these carbon emissions, 28% come from building operations. Primarily, it happens due to heating, cooling, and lighting, with energy use significantly impacted by the quality of the building envelope, especially in older buildings. The remaining 11% is just attributed to emissions from the construction process, which also includes waste, water, dust, as well as greenhouse gas emissions.[1]

Similarly, every year, 1.5 trillion bricks are produced, and while it may seem harmless, it is actually more harmful to the environment. That's right, the polluting kilns contribute to 20% of global black carbon emissions, which isn't a small number by any means. These kilns are mostly concentrated in Central and South Asia, with transportation further amplifying these emissions.

On the same measure, fine particulate matter (PM2.5/PM10) is released from the combustion of fuels in buildings, as well as in transport, especially in cities. This highlights the need for sustainable urban planning to minimize air pollution. Building construction can also release toxic dust, such as silica and hardwood dust, which are carcinogenic and can cause cancer.

---

1. Air quality in the built environment - World Green Building Council. (2022, August 17). World Green Building Council. https://worldgbc.org/healthy-equity-resilience/air-quality-in-the- built-environment/

Hydrofluorocarbons, also known as HFCs, are used for air- conditioning and refrigeration purposes. These chemicals are up to 1,000 times more dangerous than CO2 itself and contribute significantly to global warming. Their use is growing by 8-15% on an annual basis due to population growth and growing urbanization, and it is expected to rise further as the climate warms up. As 2.3 billion people worldwide are expected to purchase air conditioners or fridges soon, the demand for inefficient and high-emission appliances will surely increase.

In the developing world, residential energy use, including traditional cookstoves, open fires, and kerosene lamps, accounts for up to 58% of all global black carbon emissions. These short-lived climate pollutants can warm the atmosphere tens to thousands of times more than CO2 ever can, even though they remain in the atmosphere for a shorter period of time. Energy poverty affects a little over 1 billion people worldwide, emphasizing the need for sustainable development to tackle both energy access and emissions.

Final Word

We cannot deny the efficacy of HVAC systems. However, when used with traditional ventilation, an HVAC system can deliver fully. When it comes to CO2 accumulation within the living space, it is important for us to understand that it is a thick and dense greenhouse gas, which is heavier than air.

As a result, it tends to sink. With most HVAC systems,

the ventilation systems are placed on the ceilings, which makes it almost impossible for them to get rid of CO2 at ground level.

When this happens, the CO2 remains trapped inside, exposing the occupants to its harmful impacts. This is where we need to resort to windows and ventilation fans. The trick is to strike a balance.

CHAPTER 5
CRITICAL PERIODS IN EARLY BRAIN DEVELOPMENT

It is important for us to understand that a human being is born with a billion neurons. However, not all of them are connected. This is where the individual and those around them, including parents and other caregivers, come into the picture. Your experiences and interactions with others are responsible for making those important connections.

According to research, from the time a person is born to the age of three, these pathways come into being. As a result, the child is able to absorb valuable pieces of information while becoming accustomed to new environments.[1]

So, where does it all begin? Well, while the babies may seem like weak and helpless little beings, their brains are rapidly changing and may work overtime. These changes are what compel a child to giggle, form words, try to talk,

---

1. ZERO TO THREE. (2025, February 27). Why 0-3? | ZERO TO THREE. https://www.zerotothree.org/why-0-3/

walk, and run. This may seem a little far-fetched, but a baby's brain is capable of creating millions of brand-new connections during the first few formative years of their lives. This means that the human brain is the most flexible during the first three years of life.

Before moving forward, take a look at some of these amazing brain facts. This may seem strange, but a baby's brain has all the brain cells the baby will ever need during their lifetime. Furthermore, the size of the brain tends to double during the first year of life. Moreover, by age three, the human brain has already reached 80% of the size of a fully grown.

Also, by age two or three, the human brain has twice as many synapses as it will ever have during adulthood. After the child crosses the three-year mark, these connections become slower. It happens due to a process referred to as pruning. However, the slowing down of connections makes the brain more efficient, and by the time the child reaches the age of five, almost 90% of their brain is done growing.

Nature vs. Nurture

You must remember that the early brain development of a baby is heavily impacted by genetics. That's right. Their genes tend to form neurons while taking care of the basic wiring of the brain. However, it is important for us to understand that genes alone won't do the trick. The brain tends to adjust and adapt based on the environment it is surrounded by.

Whatever we tell our children and the things they

absorb from their environment tend to result in neural activity. For example, every time you sing a song, read, or carry out a household chore, your baby will pick it up, further activating synapses. Moreover, repetition and reinforcement result in stronger synapses. On the flip side, the synapses that aren't activated tend to get weaker with time, and they are most likely to get pruned out over time.

Therefore, it is important for a baby's brain to have a safe and supportive environment that is free of abuse, neglect, and hatred. Also, the environment shouldn't have too many stressors, as it would adversely impact the baby's brain. Here are some of the things your baby's brain needs from birth until the age of three.

Nutrition

Quality nutrition plays a key role in a baby's brain development. Infants and young children who don't receive the right number of calories and protein may be prone to physical and cognitive growth problems and delays. With malnutrition leading to smaller brains and kids suffering from long-term behavioral and cognitive deficits, lack of nutrition can take its toll.

Some key nutrition tips include adequate breastfeeding, as breast milk takes care of the baby's needs and results in neurodevelopment. Furthermore, after the age of six months, babies need iron to prevent cognitive deficits, as it is necessary for oxygen transportation, as well as brain development. Similarly, whole milk, which offers necessary fats and proteins, is important for children after their first year.

Children must also be fed solid foods that offer proteins, whole grains, fruits, and vegetables, thus ensuring a well-rounded diet to support brain growth.[2]

Play Time

Play is vital for both infants and older children. It helps them explore the environment in their surroundings, test skills, make decisions, and develop situational awareness. All of these things cumulatively strengthen the circuits of the brain. Then, there are some serve-and-return interactions. These activities may include interactions like cooing or smiling back at a baby, which are beneficial in shaping brain development, while offering stress protection. These playful exchanges, which often evolve into games like peek-a-boo, help develop the brain's architecture, which further supports cognitive growth.[3]

Reading

Reading to babies is extremely important, even when

---

2. Webster, R. (2025, February 10). How does nutrition affect the developing brain? | ZERO TO THREE. ZERO TO THREE. https://www.zerotothree.org/resource/how-does-nutrition-affect-the- developing-brain/

3. Staff, P. (2024, September 26). Why do we focus on the prenatal-to-3age period?: understanding the importance of the earliest years. Prenatal-to-3 Policy Impact Center. https://pn3policy.org/resources/why-do-we-focus-on-the-prenatal- to-3-age-period-understanding-the-importance-of-the-earliest- years/

they are young enough not to understand the words. Reading to your child at an early age is key to early language development. Hearing stories adds a significant set of words to their brains, which builds the foundation for language skills, while boosting parent-child bonding. We may not realize that reading aloud in infancy and toddlerhood can result in effective vocabulary development when a child reaches school age. Reading exposes children to emotions, sounds, and, most importantly, words, which helps them learn to recognize pictures, while imitating sounds, enhancing their language and social development.[4]

Sleep

We cannot rule out the importance of sleep. Sleep is extremely important for brain growth in infants. During their first year, when they spend much time napping, neural connections and sensory memories are formed during sleep. During the first few months of a child's life, calming techniques help babies sleep, and as they grow, it is very important for parents to establish a consistent bedtime routine. According to studies, inconsistent bedtimes, especially by the age of three, can negatively impact cognitive development, which may lead to lower performance in reading, math, and spatial awareness by the

---

4. Clinic, C. (2025, March 21). The benefits of reading to babies. Cleveland Clinic. https://health.clevelandclinic.org/the-benefits-of-reading-to-babies/

age of seven. Consistent, quality sleep sets the foundation for the right brain development.[5]

Cell Growth, Migration, and Connection Formation

While we are on the topic of early brain development, we cannot rule out the process of cell growth, migration, and the formation of connections in the brain. The process known as neurodevelopment starts with the formation of new neurons. These new neurons must then migrate to their final locations within the brain.

This process starts three to four weeks after conception has taken place. When the ectoderm tends to thicken, it forms a neural plate that develops into ridges, fusing into a neural tube. This tube thickens at the end to form parts of the brain known as the hindbrain, midbrain, and forebrain.

Neurons tend to move from the inner surface of the tube to the outer surface. The neurons are guided by the radial glia, which acts as scaffolding. This migration process occurs in an "inside-out" fashion, with older neurons forming deeper brain layers and younger ones forming layers on the outside. Moreover, some neurons migrate tangentially, but what does this mean? It means that they move parallel to the brain's surface. It is important to understand that migration can be disrupted by some external factors, such as alcohol consumption or radiation,

---

5. Kelly, Y., Kelly, J., & Sacker, A. (2013). Time for bed: associations with cognitive performance in 7-year-old children: a longitudinal population-based study. Journal of Epidemiology & Community Health, 67(11), 926–931. https://doi.org/10.1136/jech-2012-202024

which can result in intellectual disabilities or even epilepsy in individuals.

Once the neuron reaches its final destination, it begins forming connections through axons and dendrites, thus enabling functions such as vision and hearing. These axons transmit certain signals, while dendrites receive them. The longest axons can extend up to some great distances, such as from the spinal cord all the way down to the toes.

These axons grow through a growth cone that explores the environment, guided by molecular cues such as netrin, semaphorin, and ephrin. Such cues help the growth cone navigate, thus directing it to its proper destination either through attraction or repulsion.

Blood Flow Patterns and Autism

With time, we have witnessed a considerable increase in autism diagnoses. Now, research is focusing on understanding the condition's neurobiology. Autism Spectrum Disorder, or ASD, affects a child's social, emotional, as well as behavioral development, and the numbers have actually tripled during the last decade and a half. Even though genetic and environmental factors are to blame for the rising cases of autism, the exact cause of ASD still remains unclear. However, some researchers at the Children's Hospital in Los Angeles have made a considerable breakthrough by linking altered brain activity to social deficits in autism.

In a study by Dr. Bradley Peterson, 44 people with ASD were compared to 66 typically-developing individuals.

These people were matched for their age, sex, as well as their level of IQ. The researchers used advanced imaging techniques, including arterial spin labeling, to measure brain blood flow and NAA levels as markers of healthy neurons. These methods provided a more comprehensive view of brain activity and structure and revealed unexpected findings.[6]

In this exercise, the team discovered enhanced blood flow, or hyperperfusion, in large quantities of white matter in individuals suffering from ASD. This was indeed surprising, as white matter is typically associated with long-range communication between brain cells, and deficits in white matter have been linked to autism. According to Peterson, this hyperperfusion could very well be a compensatory mechanism, where brain cells are working harder to overcome white matter deficiencies, which explains why some individuals with ASD function at higher levels.

The study also explored areas with high blood flow that had lower levels of NAA, which suggests fewer healthy neurons. This further supports the idea of compensation, with the brain attempting to maintain function despite impaired white matter signaling. Peterson's research is the first to connect white matter hyperperfusion, neuron health markers, as well as ASD symptoms. It offers new insights into the neurological underpinnings of ASD. This study

6. Children's Hospital Los Angeles. (n.d.). Children's Hospital Los Angeles. https://www.chla.org/blog/experts/research-and-breakthroughs/what-can-blood-flow-tell-us-about-autism

may shift the focus of autism research toward axons and their supporting cells, which are important for understanding the mechanisms of the brain's compensation.

Developmental Windows

Most children tend to develop rapidly, showcasing different skills that emerge during specific developmental windows that start from birth and go all the way to the age of fourteen. These periods tend to reflect the individual's cognitive, emotional, and physical growth stages. For instance, babies focus on sensory exploration from birth to the age of 18 months, babies focus on sensory exploration, while between the ages of 18 months and 2 years, babies begin to define their individuality, develop vocabulary, and explore their environment.

As children transition through the ages of three to five, they start learning some of the most basic concepts like numbers and letters, and between ages six and eight, they develop social lives outside the family. It is also the time when they start forming academic and athletic habits that stay with them throughout their lives.

Between the ages of nine and 11, maturity can be inconsistent in children. Between these ages, children can start thinking logically and exploring real-world tasks like cleaning the car or mowing the lawn. Then comes the onset of puberty, which takes place at ages 11 to 14. This change leads to rapid shifts in both mind and body, making emotions harder to control and daily life more unpredictable than it was before.

Despite these developmental windows, we must remember that different children progress at different rates, which is perfectly alright. Parents may often worry whether their child is on track, but there's no need to be concerned about their child being a late bloomer unless there are some evident developmental delays, which we will discuss in the next section. If these delays are observed, seeking professional help, such as therapy, may benefit the child's development and growth.

It is important to understand that throughout all these stages, parents play a key role in supporting their child's development by offering guidance, nurturing, and appropriate interventions if they think it's necessary.

Developmental Delays

What is a developmental delay? Simply put, a developmental delay takes place when a child is slower to reach specific milestones, such as speaking their first words or taking their first step, compared to their peers. Children tend to develop skills like playing, learning, speaking, and moving at different rates, and that is fine. For a child to be a little behind isn't always a problem. However, if you notice a continuous delay in how your child develops skills, things may be problematic, and seeking professional help may be your best bet.

Developmental delays can impact a child's different areas, including cognitive or thinking skills, social and emotional skills, speech and language skills, and, most importantly, motor skills. When delays impact two or more areas in a child, it's called a global developmental delay. While some of these delays may resolve with time, conditions such as autism are lifelong and don't go away by themselves.

What causes these delays? Well, some of the most common causes of developmental delays include genetic factors, premature birth, inadequate nutrition, and exposure to toxins. Early intervention services are important for helping children who experience delays. This is often done through therapies such as speech or occupational therapy, which can improve outcomes. Developmental screening is also a useful technique that helps identify delays, and timely support increases the likelihood of the child catching up to their peers in a timely fashion.

Usually, children with developmental delays can make progress with early intervention, which helps them lead happy and healthy lives going forward. While some delays may resolve on their own, others might worsen without the right kind of support. Parents can help by providing their children with a nurturing environment that includes activities that promote skill development, like playing, reading, and following routines. Early diagnosis and intervention are important.

Final Word

Remember, the first few years of a child's life are extremely important for their brain development. During this time, the foundation for cognitive, emotional, and physical growth is laid. During this time, the brain's plasticity allows for rapid connection formation, which their experiences in a nurturing environment can significantly shape a child's abilities.

The connection between genetics and the environment, along with proper nutrition, sleep, play, and parental interactions, plays a key role in this development. While the critical periods for brain growth are limited, understanding and supporting these stages can lead to healthier outcomes for children.

Early intervention is key, especially for those facing developmental delays, thus making sure they receive the necessary resources they need in order to thrive. Parents, caregivers, and communities must recognize the significance of these early years to fully support a child's development.

CHAPTER 6
THE MECHANISM OF CO2-INDUCED NEURAL DAMAGE

In the previous chapters, we have discussed the impacts of CO2 exposure on human health and, most importantly, the brain. In this section, we will explore some other areas of CO2 exposure, such as high blood viscosity, clot formation, and the impact of CO2 exposure on neural tissues.

The increase in levels of carbon dioxide, also known as hypercapnia, in the developing brain can result in cerebral vasodilation. It is a process where blood vessels become wider, which results in increased blood flow. This type of vasodilation is an essential mechanism that ensures adequate oxygen delivery to the brain, especially during times of increased metabolic demand. For example, even a small increase in CO2 concentration can result in a substantial increase in cerebral blood flow by up to 50%. This effect plays a key role in maintaining optimal brain function when metabolic activity increases.

On the flipside, reduced CO2 levels, known as hypocapnia, induce vasoconstriction, which causes the narrowing of cerebral blood vessels and a subsequent decrease in CBF. This decrease in blood flow can limit the delivery of oxygen to the brain, and if it is prolonged, it may lead to brain dysfunction or even injury. Such disturbances in blood flow can have significant consequences on brain health, especially during the sensitive periods of brain maturation.

Furthermore, elevated CO2 levels can have an indirect impact on blood viscosity. The vasodilation associated with hypercapnia can change blood flow velocity and create stress, which can influence blood cell aggregation and viscosity. While the exact impact of CO2 on blood viscosity is still not fully understood, more studies are yet to be conducted in this area. However, it is clear that such changes in circulation can lead to more physiological effects. The extent of these changes may also depend on other factors, including pre-existing medical conditions or diseases that may have an impact on blood flow.[1]

The developing brain is vulnerable to fluctuations in CO2 levels in the blood and cerebral circulation. As the brain experiences rapid changes in energy metabolism and vascular function during its developmental stages, it becomes more prone to the impacts of CO2 imbalances. According to research, elevated CO2 levels can affect cognitive function and learning abilities in developing brains, thus making it imperative to monitor these levels in

---

1. Burch, G. E., & De Pasquale, N. P. (1965). The effect of CO2 on the viscosity of whole blood. Archiv Für Kreislaufforschung, 46(1–4), 161–167. https://doi.org/10.1007/bf02120179

younger children and individuals undergoing neurological development.[2]

From a more clinical standpoint, understanding how CO2 influences cerebral circulation is important when it comes to diagnosing and managing conditions that affect brain function. They may include stroke, hypoxia, and various other developmental disorders. Monitoring CO2 levels and CBF is a key component of clinical practice, especially for patients with neurological conditions. Such insights can aid in better treatment strategies and interventions, thus ensuring optimal brain health and function.

High CO2 Conditions and Clot Formation

Now, let's change gears and discuss the impact of high CO2 exposure on clot formation. It is a fact that high CO2 levels or hypercapnia can impact blood clot formation, thus influencing the body's hemostatic process. In some cases, this may lead to hypercoagulation (increased clotting) or hypocoagulation (decreased clotting), depending on the specific context and underlying conditions.

The coagulation cascade is a series of enzymatic reactions that result in the formation of blood clots. Such reactions can be affected by factors like pH and calcium levels, both of which are impacted by CO2 levels. Elevated

2. Kiray, M., Sisman, A., Camsari, U., Evren, M., Dayi, A., Baykara, B., Aksu, I., Ates, M., & Uysal, N. (2014). Effects of carbon dioxide exposure on early brain development in rats. Biotechnic & Histochemistry, 89(5), 371–383. https://doi.org/10.3109/10520295.2013.872298

CO_2 levels can also cause acidosis, which disrupts coagulation factor activity and the availability of calcium, thus altering the formation of clots in the body.

In some scenarios, higher CO_2 levels can also contribute to hypercoagulation by increasing platelet activation and aggregation or by elevating coagulation factors. Whereas in some cases, hypercapnia may cause hypocoagulation. In these cases, coagulation factors tend to become impaired, or increased fibrinolysis occurs. For those of you who don't know, fibrinolysis is simply the breaking down of clots. Furthermore, increased CO_2 levels can lead to the formation of microclots, which are smaller clots that may affect blood flow inside the smaller vessels.

From a more clinical standpoint, these effects on clot formation can have some serious implications. Hypercoagulation can enhance the risk of a person developing thrombosis. It can cause issues like deep vein thrombosis or pulmonary embolism. On the other hand, hypercoagulation may result in an increased risk of bleeding. Such changes in blood clotting are directly influenced by the underlying causes of hypercapnia, as well as other conditions that impact the coagulation system. This makes the management of CO_2 levels crucial in patients with clotting disorders or respiratory problems.

Compromised Blood Flow and Poor Neural Tissue Development

During neural development, poor blood flow or ischemia can make it difficult for the brain to receive enough oxygen and nutrients. This can result in brain cell damage, which in some cases can be fatal for the person. As a result, neurological deficits can take place. Some common examples include problems with speech, movement, memory, or even vision.

If blood flow is blocked for any reason, it may very well lead to an ischemic stroke. Such a stroke damages brain tissue, and in some cases, it can even be fatal. Inadequate blood supply may also cause neural tube defects (NTDs) like spina bifida, with some serious abnormalities in the arterial supply that tend to disrupt neural development.

Cerebral blood flow (CBF) is important for delivering nutrients while removing wastes from the brain. A reduction in CBF can result in ischemic stroke, while excessive blood flow or hyperemia can enhance intracranial pressure while causing brain damage. It is important to understand that certain areas in the brain are more vulnerable to ischemia. These areas include the hippocampus and cerebellum. Remember, compromised blood flow can also impact the blood-brain barrier (BBB), sometimes disrupting it. It may result in swelling, ion imbalances, and neuroinflammation, which can further cause brain tissue damage.

Blood flow regulation is also affected by the cardiovascular centers in the medulla and astrocytes, which help control the dilation of the blood vessels. Poor circulation can cause peripheral neuropathy, which often causes numbness, tingling, or pain. If blood flow problems are severe or stay for extended periods, they can result in permanent nerve damage.

Why Do Conventional Treatments Fail with Developmental Interruptions?

Oftentimes, people try to handle developmental interruptions with traditional treatments, and while it may work for some people, it can only take them so far. So, why don't these treatments work with developmental issues? Let's discuss.

Developmental interruptions, like the ones caused by things such as trauma, neglect, or brainstem damage, can hinder some key processes like emotional regulation, cognitive function, and, most importantly, social skills. Such children may struggle with forming therapeutic alliances, following instructions, or engaging in treatment, especially if they lack the emotional or cognitive maturity required to apply the therapeutic skills they may learn in therapy.

Specific challenges include trauma, which impacts emotional regulation and attachment. Then, there is also neglect, which leads to developmental delays and brainstem damage, which prevents insight, making traditional therapies less effective.

To address such problems, interventions must be tailored to the child's unique developmental needs. The responsible people should also consider the child's age, their developmental stage, and the nature of the interruption they suffer from. Early intervention is crucial in addressing delays, while a multidisciplinary approach involving therapists, educators, and other professionals ensures comprehensive support.

Building strong therapeutic relationships and involving parents in the treatment process is crucial, especially as children with developmental disruptions may have a hard time trusting other people, even if they are their therapists. Additionally, addressing underlying trauma through trauma-informed therapies like mindfulness exercises, breathing exercises, cognitive behavioral therapies, and somatic experiencing can improve outcomes.

Final Word

The impacts of CO2 exposure on brain development, cerebral circulation, and clot formation represent the relationship between environmental factors and a person's neurological health. Elevated CO2 levels can impact brain functions by altering blood flow, increasing blood viscosity, and causing clot formation.

Such disruptions are particularly concerning during brain development stages, as they can affect cognitive function while increasing the risk of neurological deficits, such as those seen in strokes and neural tube defects. Furthermore, it is important to understand that developmental interruptions caused by trauma, neglect, or brainstem damage can hinder the success of conventional treatments, as the affected children may struggle with emotional regulation, cognitive processing, and social engagement.

Addressing such challenges requires early intervention strategies and a multidisciplinary approach to ensure optimal outcomes. Understanding such mechanisms is important for improving treatment strategies and mitigating the long-term effects of neural problems.

CHAPTER 7

MODERN NURSERY DESIGN: A CRITICAL ASSESSMENT

While modern nursery designs prioritize aesthetics, it is essential to ensure good ventilation to maintain healthy indoor air quality as well. Lack of ample ventilation can result in the buildup of pollutants, moisture, allergens, and all the things that negatively affect a baby's health. Proper airflow is important for creating a safe and comfortable environment for children because stagnant air can create health risks.

The significance of proper ventilation in nurseries just cannot be overstated. One of the most common health concerns that go hand in hand with poor ventilation is the accumulation of harmful pollutants. Some of the most common examples include dust, mold, pollen, and volatile organic compounds (VOCs), which usually come from furniture and cleaning products. Such pollutants can trigger allergies, respiratory issues, and other health issues in babies whose immune systems are still growing and developing.

Moreover, stagnant air can result in higher humidity levels, creating an environment conducive to mold. As insignificant as it may sound, mold is more dangerous than we think. A few mold spores can severely affect a baby's respiratory system. Proper ventilation is the answer, as it helps regulate the temperature and humidity inside the nursery, thus ensuring a comfortable environment for the child.

Another essential aspect of good ventilation is air exchange. The best thing about a well-ventilated space is that it replaces stale indoor air with fresh, clean air, which is vitally important for maintaining indoor air quality. Without this regular exchange, air can become polluted. The air may also contain moisture and allergens, leading to health concerns. Therefore, ensuring good airflow is essential to make sure a baby's overall well-being isn't compromised.

Sadly, some of the aspects of modern nursery design can unintentionally cause poor ventilation. Many contemporary designs tend to prioritize airtightness and energy efficiency, which may seem effective for reducing energy consumption, but it can limit air circulation if not planned carefully. Moreover, larger windows, while aesthetically pleasing, are sometimes placed in such a way that they hinder natural ventilation.

Another major issue lies in the use of synthetic materials in modern nursery furniture and decor items. These items release VOCs into the air, thus compromising air quality, provided the room is not properly ventilated. In addition, many modern nurseries may lack exhaust fans in bathrooms, which results in moisture buildup and compromised air quality.

There are a few things you can do to ensure proper ventilation in a nursery. One useful measure is the strategic placement of windows. By positioning your windows to maximize natural airflow and ventilation, you can help ensure the circulation of fresh air. Furthermore, installing exhaust fans inside your bathrooms and kitchens can help get rid of excess moisture and odors that cause bad air quality.

Similarly, choosing materials with low amounts of VOC for furniture, paints, and flooring can also help decrease the release of harmful chemicals into the indoor space, thus maintaining air quality. Regularly ventilating the room by opening windows for short periods each day allows fresh air to circulate and keeps the environment healthier for the kids.

For extra air purification, one can also consider using air purifiers that contain HEPA filters. These purifiers can effectively remove dust, pollen, and other allergens. Lastly, maintaining proper humidity levels by using humidifiers or dehumidifiers can help prevent mold growth, which is a major concern in indoor spaces.

CO2 Accumulation in Traditional Cribs

Apart from poorly ventilated nurseries, the cribs aren't free from pollutants, especially CO2. That's right! Traditional cribs, while designed to offer comfort and safety for children, often contain materials and designs that could pose risks, especially concerning carbon dioxide accumulation. Most cribs use padded bumpers. Such bumpers are usually made of multiple layers of fabric, often wrapped around fiberfill or other cushioned materials. The issue with padded bumpers is that even when a mesh layer is used in their design, these materials can trap exhaled carbon dioxide from the baby's breath.

When a baby lies down, especially face down or to the side, their exhaled CO2 can be trapped by the bumper's materials. Because CO2 is heavier than oxygen, it accumulates close to the baby's face, thus creating a potentially hazardous environment where the baby may breathe in a heavy concentration of CO2, which could cause respiratory distress or suffocation.

Besides feeling suffocated and distressed, prolonged exposure to CO2 can result in bigger issues. One such issue is acidosis. As the name implies, in this condition, the amount of blood may increase in the baby's blood, which may affect several organs.

Similarly, CO2 can also cause brain damage. Premature brain injuries can also take place, as well as periventricular leukomalacia (PVL) and intraventricular hemorrhage (IVH). Furthermore, CO2 exposure can also cause retinopathy of prematurity, which is a form of eye damage.

Safer Alternatives

Breathable Bumper

Some of the new cribs in the market now offer breathable mesh bumpers. These are designed for better airflow and minimized risk of CO_2 buildup. Such bumpers use materials that let air pass through them freely, thus preventing suffocation risks.

Non-Quilted Mattresses

Nowadays, you can find mattresses that are designed with open-cell foam or similar materials that increase airflow. Such mattresses may lack the plush, quilted surface, but they keep the air circulating around the baby's face, reducing the risk of CO_2 accumulation.

Mattresses with Ventilation Holes

Newer crib mattresses have ventilation holes or channels, which are designed specially to improve airflow and allow CO_2 to escape. These ventilation systems prevent the creation of gas pockets near the baby's mouth and nose.

Minimalist Bedding

This may seem a little counterintuitive, but reducing the amount of bedding in the crib, such as heavy quilts or pillows, can promote better airflow and minimize the risk of CO_2 buildup, which is detrimental to a child's health.

Improving Air Quality in Your Baby's Room

Improving air quality in your baby's room is important for ensuring a safe and healthy environment. The first thing you can do is monitor indoor air quality using a device like the IQAir AirVisual Series. These systems offer accurate measurement of pollutants such as tiny fine particles of PM2.5. As a result, you can understand the level of contamination while identifying the best actions to improve the air quality.

Another effective way to enhance air quality is by using air purifiers. The IQAir Atem Desk is a portable option designed for small spaces such as nurseries. It uses a HyperHEPA filtration system, which removes almost 99.5% of harmful ultrafine particles as small as 0.003 microns. This technology helps ensure that the air your baby breathes is free of pollutants, thus offering a cleaner environment. Moreover, the IQAir air purifiers achieve this without releasing harmful byproducts such as ozone or similar chemicals.

When it comes to furniture, it's crucial to choose non-toxic finishes and understand that not all baby furniture marketed as safe is actually free of chemicals. Make sure to avoid composite wood furniture, as it can release harmful formaldehyde as well as other volatile organic compounds like the ones we discussed above. If your budget only allows for cheaper options, leaving the furniture outdoors for a week can help reduce emissions.

Managing humidity in your baby's room is also important. High humidity can make the air harder while making mold growth easier. It can also serve as a safe haven for bacteria and yeast. To maintain the right humidity levels, consider using a dehumidifier, as we have discussed above. Make sure you clean the dehumidifier regularly to keep it functioning effectively.

Ventilating the room is another great way to improve indoor air quality. Even with an air purifier, you need to open the windows for at least ten minutes on a daily basis. This will allow fresh air to circulate in the room. If your home has a ventilation system, it should be maintained and cleaned to prevent mold and bacteria.

Older air conditioning units can contribute to poor air quality by spreading mold spores throughout the room, and this is common with window ACs, which are rare today. If you have a window air conditioner, you need to inspect it for mold growth and replace it if necessary. If you use a central air conditioning system, change the filters regularly and schedule a thorough cleaning of the system.

When remodeling or redecorating your living space, avoiding materials that release VOCs is essential. Such materials include carpeting, paints, and furniture. VOCs can linger in the air for up to two months, which can be harmful to your baby's health. If you must remodel, opt for VOC-free paints, naturally finished furniture, and carpets made from natural fibers to prevent exposure to toxins.

Pets can also affect the air quality inside your baby's room. Pet dander, consisting of dead skin cells and hair, can irritate your baby's lungs and sinuses, resulting in chronic respiratory issues that may last a lifetime. Regular grooming of pets and keeping them out of the baby's room can help reduce this risk. Moreover, washing your baby's bedding frequently will also help eliminate accumulated pet allergens inside the room.

Lastly, a HEPA filter vacuum should be used to clean the floors and furniture inside the baby's room. A HEPA-certified vacuum cleaner is capable of capturing 99.7% of airborne particulates and tiny allergens, which is important for maintaining a clean and healthy environment for the child. Regular vacuuming with a HEPA filter removes harmful particles from the room.

PART II

CHAPTER 8
RETHINKING VENTILATION: A GROUND-UP APPROACH

In the previous chapters, we discussed indoor air quality's impact on younger brains and how exposure to indoor pollutants and greenhouse gases can result in conditions like autism. When we talk about indoor air quality, it is important to understand the precautionary measures we take to keep our living spaces clean and pure. One of those measures is the use of HVAC systems.

Ideally, an HVAC system is designed to keep the indoor air clean and pollutants-free. However, we fail to realize that, in some cases, the HVAC system serves as one of the key contributors to CO2 accumulation. Why does this happen in the first place? Well, there are several reasons for this.

It is important to understand that one of the purposes of HVAC systems is the recirculation of air. However, despite this function, they don't necessarily get rid of the built-up CO2 within our living spaces. Furthermore, the poor availability of fresh air compromises ventilation, further increasing CO_2 buildup within indoor spaces. This is where CO2 sensors need to be incorporated into an existing HVAC system.

Then, there are several HVAC maintenance issues that result in CO2 buildup within the living space. It all starts with dirty or clogged filters. They affect the airflow, which compels the HVAC system to work harder than usual. As a result, more energy is consumed, which results in extra CO2 emissions.

Dirty coils are just as bad. They tend to minimize the efficiency of the system. Another reason is the leaking refrigerant. The HVAC is once again forced to work hard, which results in increased CO2 emissions.

In some cases, the thermostat is also to blame. When a thermostat is broken or poorly set, it can also lead to energy waste and CO2 emissions, which impact the quality of our indoor spaces. Other issues include fan failures, blocked vents, and electrical issues.

It is crucial to keep an eye on gas furnaces. These furnaces can release carbon monoxide, which isn't as harmful as CO2, but it is indeed a pollutant that can be circulated within our indoor spaces through the HVAC system.

Requirements for Effective CO2 Removal

When it comes to the removal of CO2 in our living spaces, there are a few considerations we need to be mindful of. First of all, ventilation can be achieved by opening the windows and doors, as well as using an HVAC system.

Then comes the monitoring part, where you keep an eye on the occupancy levels and the levels of CO2 buildup in your living space. Let's discuss this in detail.

Ventilation

Ventilation is necessary to get rid of the built-up CO2. The primary benefit of opening doors and windows is that it allows fresh oxygen to enter our indoor environment, which tends to dilute the CO2 accumulation, especially during high occupancy periods. HVAC systems can also help, provided your HVAC system has fresh air intake while the exhaust is functional enough to get rid of CO2. It is also important to be watchful of the ventilation rate. According to the HSE, the recommended rate is 10 liters per second.[1]

Control and Monitoring

By using CO2 monitors, CO2 levels can be tracked, along with the potential issues they may pave the way for. It is important to understand that CO2 levels can go up with increased occupancy. Therefore, ventilation needs to be adjusted accordingly. According to the ASHRAE Guidelines, the concentrations of CO2 indoors should be anywhere between 800 and 1000 PPM.[2]

---

1. Using CO2 monitors - Ventilation in the workplace. (n.d.). https://www.hse.gov.uk/ventilation/using-co2-monitors.htm
2. Lemon, M. (2025, February 3). CO2 safety in restaurants, bars, venues. CO2 Meter. https://www.co2meter.com/blogs/news/co2-safety-in-

Other Alternatives

One effective way to control CO2 levels can be through plants. While this isn't the only option, it can surely help. However, you will need to have a good number of indoor plants to prevent CO2 buildup. Other technologies can also come in handy, like metal-organic frameworks. These can capture the CO2 concentration in the air while reducing the need for too much natural ventilation.

Mathematical Models for Gas Behaviors and Airflow Patterns

If you want to measure the airflow and gas behaviors, you can use certain mathematical equations. These models often use partial differential equations. Such models can either be parabolic or hyperbolic. These equations can come in handy for modeling gas flow, especially in pipelines. Some of these equations are as follows.

Partial Differential Equations

There are several models that depend on PDEs to explain the continuous flow of gas. Such equations tend to capture the relationships between density, velocity, and other properties that tend to change over space and time.

---

restaurants-bars-venus#:~:text=In%20general%2C%20the%20American%20Society%20of%20Heating%2C,CO2%20levels%20be%20maintained%20below%2 01%2C000%20ppm.

Parabolic and Hyperbolic Models

These two models are used to describe the transient flow of gas. Hyperbolic models are usually more accurate, but they can prove to be intensive as far as computations are concerned. On the other hand, parabolic models are easy to solve and can easily simulate complex structures.

One-Dimensional Flow

When it comes to gas flow modeling, one of the common simplifications means assuming a one-dimensional flow. This is where the changes, pressure, and velocity remain along the line of the duct or the pipe.

Two-Phase Flows

When a gas also contains solid particles, it is called a two-phase flow. In order to explain the motion of the particles and the gas, Lagrangian and Eulerian approaches are used.

Turbulence

In many cases, the airflow isn't laminar but turbulent. Oftentimes, models tend to incorporate turbulence using tools like the Reynolds-Averaged Navier-Stokes equation. This equation tends to average out the fluctuations of the turbulent motions.

The above-mentioned models are multipurpose and can be used in engineering, ventilation system design, gas pipeline analysis, and combustion process modeling. They are also frequently used in medicine, especially when it comes to understanding airflow and its impact on the human respiratory system. They are also used in industrial processes, such as modeling the flow of gas in fluidized beds.[3]

Floor Level Ventilation

Before we move to floor ventilation techniques, it is important to understand the risks of not having adequate floor ventilation. To begin with, inadequate floor ventilation can cause moisture accumulation. But how does moisture accumulate without ventilation? Simple! When there is insufficient airflow under the floorboards, moisture from the environment gets trapped, thus creating humidity and dampness. This trapped moisture seeps into the wood, thus raising humidity levels and potentially causing damage. The lack of ventilation keeps the wood from drying out.

Remember, moisture-induced warping is the most common type of damage that results from inadequate ventilation. But how does warping occur? When the wood absorbs too much moisture, it tends to expand beyond its natural limits, thus causing the boards to bow or warp. Not only does this affect the visual appearance of your flooring,

---

3. The Reynolds-Averaged Navier-Stokes (RANS) Equations and Models. (n.d.). System Analysis Blog | Cadence. https://resources.system-analysis.cadence.com/blog/msa2021-the-reynolds-averaged-navier-stokes-rans-equations-and-models

but it also compromises the structural integrity of the flooring. Another major concern is mold growth, which thrives in damp environments. Mold growth harms the floor and causes health issues for the inhabitants, especially young children. Some of the most common health issues include respiratory problems. In some cases, prolonged exposure to moisture can also cause wood rot, jeopardizing the wood's structure and further leading to costly repairs or replacement.

Recognizing the signs of poor ventilation and moisture damage is important for preventing long-term issues. What are the indicators of poor ventilation in wood floors? Homeowners should not ignore symptoms like musty odors, which allude to mold growth, or visible mold patches on the surface. Warped or uneven floorboards are also tell-tale signs of moisture. Regular inspections and addressing these signs can prevent damage, protecting both the investment in the flooring and the health of the occupants.

Importance of Having Floor Ventilation

Good floor ventilation is important for maintaining the quality and longevity of your wood flooring, and it doesn't come cheap. So, what are the methods for ventilating your floors? Generally, ventilation systems fall into two major categories, i.e., passive and active.

As the name implies, passive systems rely on natural airflow through some vents and work well in places where air circulates freely. On the flip side, active systems use mechanical tools, such as fans, to enhance airflow, which is especially useful in circumstances where natural ventilation isn't abundant. These systems help prevent moisture buildup under the flooring, which is a key factor in avoiding issues like warping or mold growth, thereby preserving the structure and the appearance of the floor.

Understanding Subfloor Ventilation

Subfloor ventilation systems are useful in homes, especially with elevated floors. They tend to combine vents, as well as fans, to regulate the air beneath the floor, thus maintaining a balanced moisture level. By moving air, these systems help in the elimination of excess moisture, while minimizing the chances of mold growth, mildew, and structural damage that comes with it. One of their strengths is their ability to perform in varying climates, which makes them adaptable to different conditions and flooring types. The fans play a key role in keeping the subfloor area dry, as well as well-ventilated, even when the natural airflow is insufficient.

Selecting the Right System

Choosing the best ventilation system involves considering factors such as geography, regional climate, and flooring type. In areas with high humidity, active systems with fans are often the best choice. However, in areas with good airflow, passive systems are good enough. Evaluating the environmental conditions before deciding on a ventilation method is important. A well-chosen and properly installed ventilation system not only extends the life of the flooring but also plays a key role in promoting a healthier indoor space by reducing moisture-related issues.

Case Studies of Ventilation System Modification

While we are on the topic of ventilation systems, it is important for us to look at some real-life examples. These examples demonstrate how effective floor ventilation plays a vital role in protecting wood flooring from moisture damage, extending its life, and protecting the occupants against pollutants, thus protecting their health. Let's look at some case studies for a better understanding. These case studies are the result of surveys and general trends that have been observed by people researching floor-level ventilation techniques. By reviewing these, homeowners can learn practical, proven methods for preserving the condition of wooden floors, while keeping the indoor air clean and pure.[4]

---

4. Valentine, R. (2025, March 16). Why floor ventilation matters: Protect wood flooring - Ryans restoration. Ryans Restoration. https://ryansrestoration.co.uk/why-floor-ventilation-matters- preventing-moisture-damage-in-wood-flooring/

Case Study	Solution Applied:	Results:
#1: Historic Home Renovation	Subfloor ventilation system with fans.	Stopped moisture buildup, helping preserve the original wood flooring.
#2: Modern Apartment Complex	Passive ventilation approach.	Lowered humidity, preventing warping and mold development.
#3: Coastal Property	Combination of active ventilation and dehumidifiers.	Maintained good air quality and protected the floor structure.

These examples show how different ventilation methods can be used in specific climates and building types. The key takeaway in these cases is that selecting the appropriate system is important for achieving the right balance between airflow and moisture control. By implementing these and similar ventilation solutions, property owners can protect their wooden floors from moisture damage.

Final Word

It is important to understand that maintaining indoor air quality goes beyond surface-level cleanliness. It requires a deep understanding of how HVAC systems and floor ventilation contribute to or combat air pollution and moisture buildup.

As we've seen, poorly maintained HVAC systems and insufficient floor ventilation can cause increased CO2 levels, mold growth, and structural damage, all of which pose risks to both human health and the integrity of your wooden flooring.

By implementing ventilation strategies, passive or active, and utilizing tools like CO_2 monitors, property owners can create healthier indoor environments.

CHAPTER 9

CULTURAL AND GEOGRAPHIC VARIATIONS IN AUTISM RATES

With time, access to better medical facilities has resulted in an increase in global autism rates. While the numbers were always there, the increase in awareness has played a key role in early diagnoses of children suffering from ASD.

The numbers of Autism Spectrum Disorder vary globally, with China being the country with the highest rate at 2.6%, followed by South Korea and the United States. As far as the U.S. is concerned, 1 in 59 children are diagnosed with ASD.

Globally, almost 1 in 160 children are affected by ASD. This leads to considerable social and economic effects, with the lifetime cost of autism estimated at USD 1.4 million or GBP 0.8 million. However, understanding ASD prevalence allows us to identify the necessary resources, as well as support for individuals and families that are affected by the condition.

A question arises. Why do these numbers vary from one country to the next? There are several reasons: genetic, environmental, and cultural. The variation in autism rates can also be attributed to differences in diagnostic criteria, healthcare facilities, and cultural attitudes that influence the way autism is recognized and diagnosed. Some cultures may underdiagnose or misdiagnose autism due to their lack of awareness, while others may have higher rates due to better awareness and more acceptance of the problem at hand.

The disparities in autism diagnoses are also visible among racial and ethnic groups, especially in America. These differences often stem from varying access to healthcare, diagnostic resources, and prevalent cultural perceptions. Addressing such disparities while improving cultural competence in diagnosis is necessary for ensuring equitable support and services for all individuals who suffer from this condition, regardless of their background. Increased awareness and research can result in early detection and interventions, thus helping individuals with ASD lead fulfilling lives.

Autism in Traditional Communities

This may seem strange, but more traditional communities tend to have lower Autism rates. While some may attribute this reality to a lack of resources and awareness, there are other factors at play as well. It happens due to a collection of environmental, lifestyle, and social factors. While there is no definitive reason explaining this phenomenon, some hypotheses focus on the environmental influences that might play their part, such as cleaner air, better ventilation, minimizing exposure to toxins, and lifestyle factors that differ from those in urbanized, industrialized areas. Some of these factors are as follows.

Cleaner Air and Fewer Pollutants

In traditional communities, especially in rural or isolated ones, air quality is better than in urbanized areas. Air pollution has been linked to several developmental disorders, including autism. We must understand that prenatal exposure to air pollution, especially fine particulate matter (PM2.5) and similar toxic air pollutants, can increase the risk of developmental problems in children. Communities that are less industrialized and have fewer vehicles have less air pollution, contributing to reduced risk of autism.

Indigenous communities such as Native American tribes in the U.S. or the rural populations in sub-Saharan Africa generally experience cleaner air. In contrast, urban areas with high traffic, industrial output, and pollution levels have shown higher autism rates.[1]

Better Ventilation in Living Spaces

Ventilation plays a key role in maintaining a healthy indoor environment. Traditional homes, like those made

---

1. Writer, S. (2024, November 22). Air pollution linked with increased risk of autism in children | Harvard T.H. Chan School of Public Health. Harvard T.H. Chan School of Public Health. https://hsph.harvard.edu/news/air-pollution-linked-with-increased-risk-of-autism-in-children/

from natural materials like wood, mud, or stone, tend to have better ventilation than most modern buildings, which are tightly packed and lack ventilation. Moreover, modern buildings use synthetic materials with volatile organic compounds. VOCs and other indoor pollutants are associated with developmental delays and neurodevelopmental problems in children. Traditional homes built with natural materials reduce exposure to chemicals and improve overall air quality.

In rural parts of Scandinavia, where homes are mostly built with wood, ventilation is generally simpler and more effective. This starkly contrasts the sealed, energy-efficient homes that are common in urban environments, where chemical exposure is more likely to occur.

Less Exposure to Pesticides and Industrial Chemicals

Traditional agricultural practices use fewer synthetic chemicals compared to industrial farming. This also contributes to reduced autism rates. Exposure to pesticides, herbicides, and similar chemicals in the environment is linked to developmental problems. In industrialized farming, the widespread use of such chemicals in food production and farming practices tends to increase the risk of autism in children who are exposed to these chemicals prenatally or during early childhood.

In some organic farming communities in Europe or rural India, children are likely to be less exposed to such harmful chemicals than children raised in industrial farming communities.

Diet and Nutrition

Diet plays a key role in the development of the human brain, and some traditional communities have diets that are richer in whole, unprocessed foods, with fewer additives, preservatives, or artificial sweeteners commonly found in processed foods. Evidence suggests that exposure to high levels of processed foods and artificial chemicals in the diet could negatively impact neurodevelopment.[2]

In traditional Mediterranean or Asian diets, like the ones found in rural Greece or rural Japan, which have a high intake of vegetables, fish, and natural foods, there is always a protective effect against developmental disorders compared to diets in highly processed food environments.

Social Structure and Support Networks

In traditional communities, extended families and closely knit networks often play an important role in child-rearing. Social and emotional support in these settings may help minimize stress during pregnancy and early childhood. These are the factors that have been linked to lower autism rates. Stress during pregnancy and the early postnatal period is believed to have a huge impact on the neurodevelopment of the child.

In tightly knit communities, like rural Japan or certain Native American tribes, children tend to grow up in

---

2. Buka, I., Osornio-Vargas, A., & Clark, B. (2011). Food additives, essential nutrients and neurodevelopmental behavioural disorders in children: A brief review. Paediatrics & Child Health, 16(7), e54–e56. https://doi.org/10.1093/pch/16.7.e54

environments with ample family support, lesser stress, and an increased sense of belonging. This social cohesion these children are exposed to provides protective benefits, thus reducing the risk of developmental disorders such as autism.

Lower Levels of Diagnostic Bias

In traditional communities, autism may be less likely to be diagnosed. This happens due to cultural differences in the recognition of developmental disorders. In societies with limited access to healthcare or a minimal understanding of neurodevelopmental issues, autism may be underreported.

In some remote areas, such as rural villages in parts of Africa or some of the indigenous communities in the Amazon, the understanding of autism as a clinical diagnosis just may not exist, which leads to underreporting or misdiagnosis. While this doesn't necessarily allude to lower rates of autism, it does contribute to a perception of lower autism rates in certain settings.

Global Trends in Autism Diagnoses

Between the years 1990 and 2019, the global prevalence of autism increased by a staggering 39.3%, with high-income regions such as North America, Western Europe, and the Asia Pacific showing the highest prevalence rates. It is important for us to note that regions with high socio-demographic indices experienced rapid increases in numbers, which suggests that modernization factors like improved healthcare and diagnostic practices play a part in these trends.[3]

Diagnostic Criteria Revisions

The evolution of the Diagnostic and Statistical Manual of Mental Disorders (DSM) has broadened the understanding and classification of autism. For instance, the DSM-III (1980) introduced autism as a distinct developmental disorder, while the DSM-IV (1994) recognized it as a spectrum, leading to a significant increase in diagnoses. The DSM-5 (2013) further unified these categories, contributing to a continued rise in diagnosis.

Increased Awareness and Public Perception

As societies modernize, there has been a greater emphasis on mental health awareness as well as knowledge of issues related to the human brain. This shift has resulted in better recognition of autism symptoms, especially in people without intellectual disabilities, thereby increasing diagnosis rates.[4]

---

3. Li, Y., Chen, Z., Li, X., Gu, M., Xia, N., Gong, C., Zhou, Z., Yasin, G., Xie, H., Wei, X., Liu, Y., Han, X., Lu, M., Xu, J., & Huang, X. (2022). Epidemiology of autism spectrum disorders: Global burden of disease 2019 and bibliometric analysis of risk factors. Frontiers in Pediatrics, 10. https://doi.org/10.3389/fped.2022.972809
4. CNN Newsource staff. (2023, February 2). Autism diagnosis rates

Enhanced Healthcare Infrastructure

Modern healthcare systems offer improved and enhanced screening tools and more comprehensive services now, compared to what they did 20 years ago. As a result, they are able to facilitate earlier and more accurate diagnoses of autism. For example, in the UK, the introduction of the 2013 DSM-5 criteria has led to a plateau in diagnosis rates, indicating that changes in diagnostic practices can influence prevalence trends as well.[5]

Regional Case Studies

Let's look at some regional numbers in terms of autism rates.

United States of America

From the year 2000 all the way to 2022, autism diagnoses among 8-year-olds increased from 1 in 150 to 1 in 31. This is a trend attributed to improved screening facilities, expanded diagnostic criteria, and increased public awareness. In 2025, the U.S. Department of Health and

---

have tripled in the last 16 years, new study says. https://www.alaskasnewssource.com. https://www.alaskasnewssource.com/2023/02/02/autism-diagnosis- rates-have-tripled-last-16-years-new-study-says/?

5. Bent, C. A., Barbaro, J., & Dissanayake, C. (2016). Change in autism diagnoses prior to and following the introduction of DSM-5. Journal of Autism and Developmental Disorders, 47(1), 163–171. https://doi.org/10.1007/s10803-016-2942-y

Human Services also carried out studies to explore environmental factors that contributed to this rise.

United Kingdom

Between 1998 and 2018, autism diagnoses surged by 787%, a change largely due to advancements in diagnostic practices, increased service availability, and heightened public awareness, particularly among women.[6]

Israel

From 2007 to 2018, the collective incidence of autism in children spiked from 0.46% to 1.30%. The most considerable rise was observed in toddlers and children who were attending preschool. This trend occurred despite the adaptation of DSM-5 criteria and regulatory changes that affected the eligibility for autism-related services, thus suggesting that modernization factors beyond diagnostic criteria contributed to such an increase.[7]

---

6. Russell, G., Stapley, S., Newlove-Delgado, T., Salmon, A., White, R., Warren, F., Pearson, A., & Ford, T. (2021b). Time trends in autism diagnosis over 20 years: a UK population-based cohort study. Journal of Child Psychology and Psychiatry, 63(6), 674–682. https://doi.org/10.1111/jcpp.13505
7. Davidovitch, M., Slobodin, O., Weisskopf, M. G., & Rotem, R. S. (2020). Age-Specific Time Trends in incidence rates of Autism Spectrum Disorder following adaptation of DSM-5 and Other ASD-Related Regulatory Changes in Israel. Autism Research, 13(11), 1893–1901. https://doi.org/10.1002/aur.2420

Sleeping Practices, Infant Care, and Autism Rates

Sleeping Arrangements: Co-sleeping vs. Independent Sleeping

In regions and cultures where co-sleeping is common, such as Japan, India, and some major parts of East Asia, infants often share a bed or a room with their parents for an extended period until they reach a certain age. Within these settings, behaviors such as frequent night waking or dependency at bedtime are often seen as normal elements of early childhood. As a result, early signs of autism, like irregular sleep patterns or lack of independent sleeping habits, may be overlooked or interpreted as typical behavior, as per the culture. This normalization can result in a delay in identifying developmental disparities that come with autism.

Conversely, in cultures with independent sleeping practices, such as in the United States, as well as some parts of Western Europe, there is often a greater emphasis on infants sleeping in their own beds or even their own rooms. In these contexts, disruptions in a child's sleep patterns or disengagement may stand out more clearly. This cultural emphasis on independence in sleep can help parents and healthcare providers observe atypical behaviors much sooner, potentially resulting in earlier autism diagnoses.

Parenting Style and Expectations

Cultural attitudes toward parenting also play a key role

in the way autism-related behaviors are perceived. In collectivist cultures, like those in China and some parts of the Middle East, there is a strong emphasis on interdependence within the family. Children who are shy, quiet, or reserved may be seen as well-behaved or modest, and overt parental involvement in daily activities is seen as the norm. Such cultural values sometimes tend to obscure the signs of autism. These signs may include reduced eye contact or limited social interaction. In those cultures, such traits are not necessarily viewed as problematic within the cultural context. As a result, early detection of autism may not be possible.

Alternatively, individualist cultures like those in the U.S., UK, and Australia place special emphasis on independence, verbal expression, and social engagement. Children are often encouraged to assert themselves and interact openly with other people. Within these cultures, deviations from expected developmental milestones, like a lack of verbal communication or eye contact, are more likely to raise concerns among the parents and loved ones. Parents and educators in these societies are quicker in initiating developmental screening, which can result in higher and earlier autism diagnosis rates.

Healthcare Access and Awareness

Access to healthcare and awareness of developmental problems are critical factors that tend to intersect with cultural norms to influence autism diagnosis. In modern or urbanized regions, regardless of culture, there is generally better access to pediatric care, developmental screenings, and, most importantly, specialized diagnostic services. Public health initiatives, increased media exposure, and broader professional training tend to contribute to greater awareness of autism, which further results in more frequent and earlier diagnoses.

On the other hand, in less-developed areas or in more traditional settings, autism may be underdiagnosed or even misdiagnosed. Limited access to healthcare facilities, a shortage of trained professionals, and prevailing stigmas surrounding developmental disorders can all contribute to diagnostic issues. In some scenarios, parents may attribute their child's atypical behaviors to spiritual beliefs, family stressors, or temporary developmental phases rather than seriously thinking about medical explanations such as autism.

CHAPTER 10

ARCHITECTURAL SOLUTIONS FOR HEALTHIER ENVIRONMENTS

From air quality and physical comfort to mental and physical well-being, the indoor environment has a key impact on human health. As urbanization continues to grow and modernization seeps into our day-to-day lives, understanding how architectural solutions can optimize these aspects is extremely important. Let's explore the intersection of architecture and health, while detailing important strategies focusing on improving air quality, enhancing comfort, and promoting overall well-being.

In the following sections, we will take a look at some of the latest research in building design, the role of building materials in health, and some of the most innovative approaches to energy efficiency that do not compromise the health of occupants.

Architectural Specifications for Health-Optimized Building Design

Spatial Layout and Proportions

- Building Design: The design of a building must follow spatial configuration as the top priority, as it encourages healthy air circulation, accessibility to natural light, as well as ease of movement. Several specifications are essential to make sure they deliver optimal health outcomes.
- Ceiling Heights: This may seem insignificant, but it is important. The minimum recommended ceiling height in residential areas is 2.7 meters, which equates to 8.9 feet. This results in better air circulation, thus minimizing the risk of airborne contaminants accumulating inside the living space. Higher ceilings in common areas that are 3.5 meters or 11.5 feet in commercial and public buildings encourage vertical airflow, which facilitates the dissipation of pollutants, thus keeping the indoor space clean and healthy.[1]
- Room Dimensions: The volume of interior

1. EFFECT OF CEILING HEIGHT ON THE NATURAL VENTILATION OF AN "INFINITE" SCREENHOUSE: MODEL PREDICTIONS | International Society for Horticultural Science. (n.d.). https://www.ishs.org/ishs- article/1037_41

spaces is crucial for indoor air quality. An ideal room should have at least 20 cubic meters of air per occupant to make sure there is sufficient air exchange. However, for office spaces, the recommended density is one person per 10 to 12 square meters to maintain the right amount of ventilation.

- Window-to-Floor Ratio: In order for us to optimize natural ventilation, the window-to-floor area ratio should ideally be anywhere between 1:8 and 1:10. This allows for sufficient airflow and some light penetration. Windows should also be in perfect working condition to provide occupants control over ventilation.[2]

Lighting and Daylighting

Natural light plays an important role in maintaining what we refer to as circadian rhythms. These have been shown to directly impact sleep patterns, as well as a person's overall mental health. A key guideline in architectural design is the incorporation of daylighting strategies in order to minimize dependence on artificial lighting while enhancing the well-being of the occupants. The optimal daylight factor is around 2-5%, which offers a

---

2. Isaacs, N. P. (2024). 'The window area shall be at least one-tenth of the area of the room': The origins of a daylight (and ventilation) requirement in modern building codes. Lighting Research & Technology, 56(6), 637–659. https://doi.org/10.1177/14771535231225363

considerable amount of lighting during the day while reducing glare and heat buildup.[3]

- Window Orientation and Shading: Windows should be oriented to increase exposure to sunlight while reducing direct glare and excessive heat. South-facing windows in the Northern Hemisphere and north-facing windows in the Southern Hemisphere are the ideal configurations for passive solar gains in winter and minimizing heat during summer.
- Light Intensity: The recommended level of light intensity for living spaces is somewhere between 150 and 300 lux, while workspaces demand higher levels, which are anywhere between 300 and 500 lux, depending on the task at hand. Integrating advanced light-diffusing materials and LED lighting with adjustable color temperature allows us to balance both energy efficiency and occupant comfort.[4]

Acoustic Design

Excessive noise is one of the most common contributors to stress, sleep disturbances, and long-term

---

3. TEN Key Daylight & Electric Light Metrics. (n.d.). https://www.iesve.com/discoveries/article/3813/ten-key-daylight-and-electric-metrics
4. Kumar, M. (2023, April 12). Illuminance levels indoors: Your standard lux level chart. Prana Air. https://www.pranaair.com/blog/illuminance-levels-indoors-the-standard-lux-levels/

cardiovascular problems. Acoustic design must, therefore, be prioritized in building designs. The following specifications are crucial for minimizing noise pollution in buildings.

- Sound Insulation: Building elements like walls, floors, and ceilings must include materials that absorb sound rather than reflect it to create noise. For residential areas, a sound insulation rating of STC 50 or higher is recommended in order to prevent noise intrusion from neighboring units.[5]
- Acoustic Ventilation: Mechanical systems such as ventilation ducts and air handling units should be designed to minimize noise production. The Noise Rating scale can be used to make sure the mechanical systems do not exceed a threshold of NR-35 to prevent disturbing noise levels in sleeping and living spaces.

Building Materials and Their Effect on Air Quality and Circulation

This may seem trivial, but it is more important than you think it is. The materials used in constructing or remodeling

---

5. Surfaces, A. (2024, January 22). Understanding Sound Transmission Class (STC) rating. Acoustical Surfaces. https://www.acousticalsurfaces.com/blog/acoustics-education/sound-transmission-class-stc-rating/

your indoor space play a key role in indoor air quality. Let's look at some modern and traditional materials.

Traditional Building Materials

Historically, many building materials have been known for their durability and insulating properties, but their impacts on air quality were not always considered. Here are some traditional building materials.

- Wood: Wood is a common building material found in living and commercial spaces. It can have both positive and negative impacts on indoor air quality. While natural wood can help regulate humidity and temperature, it may also emit volatile organic compounds (VOCs), including formaldehyde, especially if the wood is treated with chemical finishes. Non-toxic and untreated wood and finishes like linseed oil or natural beeswax are safer and healthier alternatives.
- Stone and Brick: These materials are excellent for thermal mass, as they absorb and release heat very slowly. However, brick and stone also have the tendency to trap moisture, which paves the way for mold and bacteria if not properly sealed. These materials should be coupled with breathable systems that allow moisture to evaporate without accumulation for optimal health.

Modern Building Materials

As the demand for energy-efficient and healthy buildings has increased, modern materials have been developed that support air quality and energy performance. Some of these materials are as follows.

- Low-VOC Paints and Coatings: Traditional paint products tend to release VOCs. Such fumes contribute to poor indoor air quality, which further leads to respiratory problems. Today, low-VOC and zero-VOC paints, like the ones based on natural pigments, offer healthy alternatives for interior themes and color schemes.
- Bamboo and Cork: The great thing about both of these materials is that they are renewable, durable, and contain natural air-purifying properties. Bamboo, for instance, has a high cellulose content, which has the ability to absorb moisture and regulate indoor humidity. Cork is naturally fire-resistant and provides excellent acoustic insulation, thus making it ideal for both floors and walls.
- Insulation Materials: Modern insulation options like sheep wool and cellulose are made from recycled paper. Hence, they are non-toxic and offer effective thermal insulation. These materials also serve as natural air purifiers, as they absorb harmful substances from the air, which is the exact opposite of conventional

fiberglass or foam insulations that may off-gas toxic chemicals, thus compromising indoor air quality.

Strategies for Maintaining Air Quality

Considering our conversation so far, you can understand that a major concern in modern building design is indoor air quality. Building materials and ventilation systems must work together to ensure that indoor air remains clean and fresh. Some considerations for improving IAQ are as follows.

- Filtration Systems: By using HEPA filters or activated carbon filters in ventilation systems, we can significantly improve indoor air quality by removing particulate matter, allergens, and the most notorious VOCs. Such filters should be maintained regularly to ensure optimal performance.
- Moisture Control: While filtration systems are effective, moisture should also be controlled to improve indoor air quality. Excess moisture in the building envelope can result in mold growth and other microbial contaminants that affect air quality. Vapor barriers and moisture-resistant materials, such as cementitious boards or moisture-wicking insulation, can be beneficial in preventing this.

Modifications to Current Building Practices for Improved Air Quality

Integrated Natural Ventilation

Natural ventilation is extremely important for maintaining fresh air within buildings, especially in highly energy-efficient designs where airtightness can cause poor air quality, compromising the health and well-being of the occupants. Modern building designs should integrate natural ventilation strategies with mechanical systems to optimize air exchange without compromising thermal comfort or energy efficiency. Here are two ways of doing so.

- Stack Ventilation: In multi-story buildings, stack ventilation depends upon the principle of buoyancy. For those who don't know, this is where warm air rises and creates a pressure differential that pulls fresh air into lower floors. This can be achieved through strategically placed vents or openings that ensure optimal airflow.
- Cross Ventilation: As the name implies, cross-ventilation works by creating pressure differences on opposing sides of a building, thus drawing fresh air through the building. This is especially effective in open-plan spaces, and it can be enhanced through operable windows, skylights, and, most importantly, vents.

Hybrid Ventilation Systems

As the name suggests, hybrid ventilation systems combine natural and mechanical ventilation systems, such as energy recovery ventilators (ERVs) or heat recovery ventilators (HRVs). These mechanisms ensure fresh air intake while ensuring that thermal energy is conserved. Hybrid systems offer several benefits. To begin with, these systems minimize the load on mechanical heating and cooling systems, which helps save energy. Secondly, these systems offer controlled air from outside, thus keeping the humidity and the pollutants at bay.

Smart Ventilation Controls

With rampant advancements in smart technology, new ways of optimizing ventilation are coming up. Sensors can detect CO2 levels, humidity, and pollutants in indoor spaces, thus adjusting the ventilation accordingly. Demand-controlled ventilation (DCV) can be integrated into the HVAC system, thus ensuring that air quality is maintained without any excessive energy use.

Final Word

Creating a healthy indoor environment through thoughtful architectural solutions is important for promoting the occupants' physical and mental well-being. From optimizing air quality with natural ventilation strategies and selecting building materials that promote a healthier atmosphere to enhancing comfort through lighting and acoustic design, each and every element of building design plays a key role.

As urbanization grows, incorporating health-optimized strategies into new and existing buildings will improve the quality of life for occupants and contribute to the sustainability of urban spaces. By prioritizing health-conscious design practices, we can create environments that nurture the body and the mind, ensuring a more sustainable and comfortable future.

CHAPTER 11
THE SCIENCE OF SLEEP ENVIRONMENTS

Sleep is extremely important for both physical and cognitive development, especially during infancy. A child's sleep environment influences the quality and duration of their rest, and it can also profoundly impact their overall health and brain development. During the last few decades, research into sleep environments has been extensive, with special emphasis on factors like quality, room temperature, and sleeping posture.

In the following paragraphs, we will take a deep dive into the science of infant sleep patterns, with a special focus on how sleep environments and relevant factors like CO2 accumulation, ventilation, and design. We will also look at how these factors can impact a child's brain development and overall health and well-being. We will also explore some effective and practical strategies for creating optimal sleep spaces that help ensure safety, comfort, and proper ventilation.

Infant Sleep Patterns and Brain Development

It is a fact that infants' sleep patterns are different from those of their adult counterparts, largely due to the rapid growth and development in their brains and bodies. Newborn babies tend to spend a significant chunk of their sleep in what we call the Rapid Eye Movement (REM) sleep, which is a crucial process for brain development. REM sleep is associated with several other important processes like memory consolidation, learning, and emotional regulation, all of which are crucial for early brain development.

A typical newborn may sleep anywhere between 14 and 17 hours on a daily basis. However, this sleep is broken into multiple periods throughout the day and night. As the baby grows, the number of sleep periods tends to decrease, and the amount of time spent in REM sleep goes up. By the time they are 6 months old, babies typically sleep anywhere between 12 and 14 hours per day, with a greater proportion of that sleep occurring at night, which allows for extended periods of uninterrupted REM sleep.

However, the quality of this sleep is not solely determined by how long a child sleeps. Sleep environments also play a key role in ensuring that babies achieve the deep, restorative sleep that is extremely necessary for proper brain development. Studies have revealed that sleep disturbances, whether they are caused by noise, temperature, or poor air quality, can significantly impact neural development and cognitive outcomes later in life.

CO_2 Accumulation and Sleep Environments

One of the crucial factors in sleep environments for children is the buildup of carbon dioxide within the sleeping area. CO_2 is produced naturally when a human breathes, and it is expelled from the room through ventilation or air circulation. However, in tightly packed spaces or poorly ventilated rooms, CO_2 levels can go up to unhealthy levels, especially during sleep hours when breathing is deeper and more consistent among the occupants.

Research suggests that elevated CO_2 levels during sleep can have dangerous impacts on cognitive performance, as well as general well-being. In infants, high CO_2 concentrations may cause disrupted sleep, shallow breathing, and even an increased risk of Sudden Infant Death Syndrome, but that is absolutely rare. According to a study published in the Journal of Applied Physiology, infants sleeping in rooms where CO_2 levels are higher than 1000 ppm experienced reduced oxygen levels in their blood, which could impact brain function and sleep quality.[1]

The Impact of Sleep Environment on CO_2 Levels

- Traditional Cribs: In a traditional crib,

---

1. News-Medical. (2020, April 21). Atmospheric CO2 levels can cause cognitive impairment. https://www.news-medical.net/news/20200421/Atmospheric-CO2-levels-can-cause- cognitive-impairment.aspx

especially when the crib is enclosed by a bumper or placed in a poorly ventilated room, CO_2 buildup is highly likely to occur. The baby's own exhaled CO_2 may also linger in the space around them if the room is not adequately ventilated. In addition, if the baby sleeps on a soft mattress or is covered by heavy bedding, these factors can contribute to CO_2 buildup by restricting the flow of air in the baby's surrounding areas.

- Co-sleeping Setups: Co-sleeping, also known as bed-sharing, is another common sleep arrangement, particularly in Eastern contexts. While co-sleeping can offer benefits like easier nighttime feeding, it also paves the way for the risk of CO_2 accumulation where the baby sleeps. In a smaller space, like a parent's bed, the concentration of CO_2 can rise at a staggering pace, especially if both the parent and the child are breathing in close proximity to one another.
- Modified Designs: Newer crib designs that ensure better airflow and better ventilation have been shown to minimize CO_2 accumulation in babies' sleeping spaces. A common example is baby cribs with mesh sides or those that are placed in rooms with higher airflow, such as near open windows or air vents. Furthermore, some modern bassinets are designed with a built-in ventilation system to maintain air

circulation for as long as the baby sleeps during the night.

The Importance of Nighttime Ventilation

The right amount of ventilation during sleep is important for maintaining a safe and healthy sleep environment for babies. Proper ventilation helps regulate temperature and humidity while removing excess CO_2 and other gases. Without the right amount of airflow, a room can become stale, with rising levels of carbon dioxide that can interfere with the quality of sleep, while considerably impacting the baby's brain growth.

Strategies for Maintaining Air Quality During Sleep

Ensure Room Ventilation:

Air circulation can be achieved by something as simple as opening windows or using a fan in the room. However, the fan should not be blowing directly on the baby to avoid discomfort or possible respiratory problems. Direct exposure to cold air can also cause congestion. If outdoor air quality is poor in your locale, an air purifier with a HEPA filter can come in handy. Some models also come with a CO_2 sensor to provide real-time monitoring of air quality inside the baby's room.

Monitor CO2 Levels:

Investing in a CO_2 monitor is a simple yet effective

way to ensure the room has the right amount of air exchange. Ideally, CO2 levels should not go beyond 1000 ppm. The lower the number is, the better off you will be, and so will the baby. Using a room thermometer with a humidity sensor can also help maintain the right air quality. A humidity level between 50% and 60% is ideal for preventing mold growth and maintaining comfort.[2]

Positioning the Crib:

Do not make the mistake of placing the cribs in corners or up against walls where the airflow is scarce. However, you must position the crib near an open window or in the middle of the room for better air circulation.

Climate Control:

Maintaining a stable room temperature of around 68-72°F or 20-22°C is just perfect for infants. If the baby's room is too hot or too cold, it can disrupt sleep while contributing to overheating or hypothermia, both of which have been linked to an increased risk of SIDS, which we discussed a few paragraphs ago. In areas with extreme temperatures, air conditioning or heating can help regulate

2. Gutierrez, J. (2025, March 17). Managing ideal indoor humidity level to prevent mold growth | GP inspections. Guaranteed Property & Mold Inspection. https://www.gpinspect.com/article/humidity-level-to- prevent-mold/

room temperature, but it's important to ensure that the airflow is directed away from the crib.[3]

Creating Optimal Sleep Environments: Balancing Safety, Comfort, and Ventilation

When designing a sleep environment for your baby, safety, comfort, and proper ventilation should be the primary considerations. The rest are secondary. Here are some detailed guidelines to create an optimal environment where the baby is safe and at peace.

Safety First:

- Firm Mattress: A firm and flat mattress provides the safest sleeping surface for infants, as soft mattresses can enhance the risk of suffocation or SIDS.
- Avoiding Soft Bedding: Make sure you avoid pillows, blankets, and stuffed animals in the crib, as these can result in a suffocation hazard. Sleep sacks or wearable blankets are safer alternatives for keeping the baby warm and safe.
- Safe Sleep Position: Infants should always be placed on their backs to sleep, as this minimizes the risk of SIDS. A firm mattress that is free of pillows or other items supports this safe sleep position for the child.

---

3. WebMD Editorial Contributor. (2023, April 15). What's the right room temperature for a baby? WebMD. https://www.webmd.com/baby/what-is-the-right-room-temperature-for-a-baby

Comfort:

- Temperature Control: A room temperature between 68- 72°F is ideal for an infant. Too much warmth can cause overheating, compromising the child's comfort and keeping them from breathing properly.
- Noise Considerations: While there are some white noise machines that may help soothe babies, excessive noise can actually disrupt sleep patterns. It is best to avoid loud or jarring sounds during sleep time. Low-volume white noise or the sound of a fan can help mask sudden disturbances that may affect the child's sleep.
- Lighting: Darkness is important for promoting good sleep in children. Therefore, you must consider blackout curtains to help keep the room dark during naps or nighttime sleep. It is important because darkness helps us release melatonin, the hormone that is responsible for sleep regulation.

Proper Ventilation:

- Window Positioning: If possible, make sure to keep windows slightly open to allow fresh air to enter and circulate. However, be mindful of the quality of the outdoor air.

- Air Purifiers: If necessary, try investing in an air purifier with a CO_2 sensor to monitor and regulate the air quality in the room where the baby sleeps.
- Humidity Control: Make sure to keep the humidity in the room somewhere between 40-60%. Too much humidity can also cause discomfort, contributing to respiratory issues. Too little humidity can backfire, drying out the baby's skin and airways, which are instrumental in breathing.

Final Word

Creating an appropriate sleep environment is important to ensure that infants sleep safely and develop and grow properly. The quality of sleep significantly influences brain development, physical growth, and overall well-being, and the environment in which the baby sleeps plays an essential role in this.

By effectively understanding the science of sleep, CO_2 accumulation, and the importance of ventilation, parents and caregivers can make informed decisions about how to design a safe, comfortable, and ventilated space for their children. Proper attention to such factors can result in healthier sleep patterns, better brain development, and a reduced risk of sleep-related health problems.

CHAPTER 12
PRACTICAL PREVENTION STRATEGIES FOR PARENTS

Ensuring good ventilation, especially in the early years of your child's life, is crucial for maintaining a healthy indoor environment. The right amount of airflow helps lower the levels of airborne pollutants, allergens, and microorganisms on the inside. Such practices support the overall well-being of children and other occupants. While awareness of ventilation has considerably increased in recent years, the underlying principles remain essential for general health and the prevention of infections in young children's spaces.

Authorities like the Health and Safety Executive (HSE) and the Department for Education (DfE) recommend that all occupied areas in early years settings be properly ventilated without compromising the comfort of learning and play environments. All this can be achieved through both mechanical and natural ventilation mechanisms. Mechanical systems should be optimized to allow more fresh air to enter, and they must be checked regularly to make sure they meet current standards. Ideally, such systems should run on full fresh air intake whenever feasible, especially when they are confined to a single room and supplemented with outdoor air.

Natural ventilation techniques like opening windows play a key role as well. In areas that experience cooler weather, windows can be left slightly open to allow continuous background ventilation and also to refresh the indoor air. Adjustments like opening high-level windows can help reduce drafts, and making changes to furniture arrangements may further support comfort by limiting direct exposure to colder air.

In order to maintain a warm and comfortable space while enhancing ventilation, several practical strategies can be utilized. Increasing the airflow when rooms are unoccupied, allowing children to wear extra layers indoors, and effectively using heating systems without blocking vents are some important considerations we can be mindful of. In colder conditions, using small, consistent ventilation openings like trickle vents may be preferable to bigger openings that rapidly tend to cool the room. Dressing children appropriately for varying temperatures also supports their comfort levels.

With time, CO2 monitors have become common tools in early years environments as a way to monitor air quality. Elevated carbon dioxide levels allude to the fact that the space may need improved ventilation. By making good use of CO2 monitors, the occupants can more easily identify areas where airflow needs to be enhanced. When levels exceed the recommended limits, increasing ventilation can help ensure better and healthier air quality, while ensuring a better environment for young children.

Daily Routines and Practices that Can Help Maintain Optimal Air Quality

For us to ensure optimal indoor air quality, it's essential to adopt a holistic approach that integrates consistent daily practices, regular maintenance, and awareness of external environmental factors. These things include everything from ventilation and cleaning to mindful product usage, while staying informed about outdoor pollution levels. By regularly checking your Air Quality Index (AQI) using resources like AirNow.gov, you can tailor your routines and actions to current air quality conditions, promoting a healthier indoor environment for everyone.[1]

Daily Routines and Practices

Ventilation:

To improve the air quality of your living space, it's crucial to allow fresh air to enter. Open windows and doors for as much as 15- 30 minutes every day, especially when the indoor air feels stagnant or if the pollution levels are higher than usual. This helps to expel accumulated pollutants, moisture, and CO2, thus refreshing the indoor

---

1. AQI Basics | AirNow.gov. (n.d.). https://www.airnow.gov/aqi/aqi-basics#:~:text=When%20AQI%20values%20are%20above,also%20has%20a%20specific%20color.

environment. On days when outdoor air quality is good, opening windows more frequently can be extremely beneficial.

Cleaning:

Dust and allergens can also build up quickly, especially on carpets, rugs, and upholstered items. Regular cleaning with a vacuum cleaner equipped with a HEPA filter will help remove dust, pet dander, and other particles that can degrade air quality. Moreover, wiping down surfaces frequently can prevent the buildup of dust and prevent it from being disturbed through the air. The use of non-toxic and low-emission cleaning products further minimizes exposure to harmful chemicals.

Air Purifier:

Using an air purifier with a HEPA filter can considerably enhance indoor air quality, especially in higher-traffic areas. Such purifiers effectively capture fine particles of dust, pollen, pet dander, and airborne allergens and pollutants. Make sure the air purifier is of the right size for the room it's placed in, and run continuously in areas with poor ventilation or higher pollutant levels.

Ventilation Schedule:

Besides opening windows, creating a schedule for ventilation is key. Opening windows for several minutes in the morning and repeating the same in the evening can help flush away any buildup of indoor air contaminants. This is particularly helpful when the outdoor air quality is favorable, which allows for the exchange of stale indoor air with fresh outdoor air. If you live in a locale with rapid temperature changes, ventilating during the warmer parts of the day can help maintain comfort.

Product Usage:

When shopping for cleaning or other household products that can emit strong fumes, it's essential to ensure the right amount of ventilation. Opening windows or using a fan to help clear the air of potentially harmful chemicals can be handy. This is especially true when using products such as paints, varnishes, or aerosol cleaners that release volatile organic compounds (VOCs), which can adversely affect health.

Indoor Plants:

Certain indoor plants, like spider plants, peace lilies, and aloe vera, can naturally purify the air. These plants can absorb harmful toxins, while releasing oxygen, thus creating a healthier indoor environment. Regular care is important in order to maintain their air-purifying capabilities, so make sure to water and dust your plants frequently to keep them healthy and functional.

Humidity Control:

Humidity levels also play a crucial part in maintaining indoor air quality. The air can become excessively dry in dry environments, irritating the respiratory system. Using a humidifier helps maintain balanced humidity levels, particularly during the winter when indoor heating systems dry out the air. However, it is important to be mindful not to over-humidify, as excess moisture can cause mold growth.

Outdoor Exercise:

Before indulging in outdoor physical activities, it is important to check the AQI for your area. On days when pollution levels are high, consider adjusting your routine to avoid exposure to harmful outdoor air. If pollution is higher than usual, try indoor exercises like yoga or aerobics, or opt for activities in areas with better air quality, like parks with lots of greenery.

Reduce Car Use:

Reducing car usage helps cut down on vehicle emissions that cause poor air quality. These emissions can enter our living space, thus affecting our health. Walking, biking, or carpooling are some of the most sustainable alternatives that not only reduce air pollution but also keep your health in good shape. Using public transportation is another effective way to minimize your carbon footprint, while reducing traffic-related pollution.

Fuel Vehicle Strategically:

When refueling your vehicle, make sure to do it when ozone levels are typically lower, such as early in the morning or late in the evening. During these times, the air is cooler, and pollution levels tend to be less extreme, which reduces the environmental impact of fueling.

Specific Schedules and Procedures

Air Purifier Maintenance:

Regular maintenance of the air purifier is important for ensuring its effectiveness. Follow the manufacturer's recommendations for filter replacement. This must happen every 6-12 months, depending on the usage. If you notice reduced airflow or an increase in allergies or asthma symptoms, chances are it is time to change the filter.

Cleaning Schedule:

Establish a regular cleaning routine to prevent dust accumulation, dirt buildup, and allergens. Make sure to clean surfaces, carpets, and upholstery at least once a week using low-emission cleaning products. This cleaning routine will help minimize the buildup of harmful particles in your living space, while promoting a healthier living environment.

Ventilation Schedule:

A ventilation schedule should be part of your routine.

Opening windows for a few minutes in the morning and evening, especially on days with good outdoor air quality, helps you maintain fresh air exchange without a considerable drop in indoor temperature. Be mindful of the weather and adjust ventilation duration to maintain comfort.

HVAC Maintenance:

Your heating, ventilation, and air conditioning systems play a key role in maintaining good indoor air quality. Make sure to schedule regular maintenance for your HVAC system, which includes cleaning and replacing filters, while ensuring that the ventilation system is functioning properly. Regular checks help prevent the buildup of dust and mold within the ducts. It also helps ensure clean and efficient airflow throughout your indoor space.

Indoor Plant Care:

Taking care of your indoor plants is important to maintaining air quality inside the house. Make sure to dust and water your plants regularly to keep them in top shape. Healthy plants will continue to purify the air by absorbing toxins and releasing oxygen, which further leads to a better atmosphere inside your home.

Radon Testing:

Pay attention to this one. Radon is a naturally occurring

radioactive gas, and it can build up in enclosed spaces, posing serious health risks. In areas known for high radon potential, testing radon levels in your home is important. If the radon levels are high, take immediate steps to minimize exposure. You can do things like sealing cracks in floors and walls or installing a radon mitigation system.

Mold and Mildew Prevention:

Mold and mildew can live and grow in damp environments, and they significantly impact indoor air quality. To prevent mold growth, make sure you address any moisture issues in your home, such as leaks or excess humidity. You can use dehumidifiers, fix leaks, and ensure proper ventilation in areas like bathrooms and basements. It can help keep mold and mildew at bay, thus promoting a healthier indoor environment. Remember, mold and mildew affect not only your health but also that of your children. It also affects the structural integrity of your house.

CO2 Monitoring

In order to monitor CO2 levels in your home, you can use a dedicated CO2 monitor or an air quality monitor, including a CO2 sensor. Such devices offer real-time readings, and many of the models available in the market can send alerts when CO2 levels exceed a threshold. Understanding typical CO2 levels and their fluctuations based on different factors, like occupancy, activities, and ventilation, can allow you to better manage your indoor air quality.

When choosing a device to monitor CO2 levels, you have two main options i.e., dedicated CO2 monitors and air quality monitors. Dedicated CO2 monitors are designed to measure CO2, and most of them often come with additional features like data logging and alerts. Some air quality monitors include CO2 sensors alongside sensors for other pollutants and environmental factors, offering a holistic view of your indoor air quality.

The placement of the monitor is key to ensuring accurate readings. Ideally, it should be positioned in a central place within the room. This place should be away from windows, doors, and vents, and at least two meters away from any potential CO2 source, like open flames. Moreover, placing the monitor at head height, somewhere between 1 and 2 meters off the ground, helps ensure that it measures the air you are breathing rather than air near the floor or the ceiling, where CO2 may not be concentrated enough.

Proper calibration and maintenance are important for obtaining correct readings from your CO2 monitor. Always make sure to follow the manufacturer's instructions for setup as well as upkeep. It's also vital to take regular readings, especially during times when the room is heavily occupied, as CO2 levels can fluctuate throughout the day.

As far as interpreting the readings is concerned, CO2 levels between 400 and 1000 parts per million are generally considered acceptable for indoor environments. If levels go beyond 1000 ppm, this may allude to the fact that the space is poorly ventilated and needs more fresh air to lower the CO2 concentration. CO2 levels can rise due to increased occupancy, increased physical activity, or using combustion appliances like stoves or heaters, all of which release ample amounts of CO2 into the air.[2]

If you notice consistently high CO2 levels, taking action for better ventilation is important. One simple approach is to open the windows or to use exhaust fans for fresh air. While air purifiers can improve air quality by getting rid of particles and gases, they do not remove CO2, so increasing ventilation is usually the most effective means to minimize CO2 levels. In more serious cases, you might consider using a whole-house ventilation system that can continuously bring fresh air into your home, further improving the air quality.

Final Word

Prioritizing practical strategies, from ensuring consistent ventilation and maintaining cleaning routines to making informed and educated choices about household products and monitoring air quality using tools like CO2 monitors and awareness of the outdoor AQI, forms a strong defense against indoor air pollutants.

By integrating these daily habits and ensuring recommended maintenance schedules, parents can cultivate

---

2. Kane International. (n.d.). What are safe levels of CO and CO2 in rooms? | Kane International Limited. Kane International Limited. https://www.kane.co.uk/knowledge-centre/what-are-safe-levels-of- co-and-co2-in-rooms

healthier living spaces for their children, which helps them ensure their well-being while laying the foundation for a healthier future.

CHAPTER 13

ECONOMIC IMPLICATIONS OF THE AUTISM CRISIS

Navigating the financial side of autism treatment can be extremely overwhelming for families. The average cost tends to vary, and it is influenced by the type and intensity of therapy, where the family lives, and the individual needs of the child suffering from autism. These factors all collectively contribute to the overall cost, while making it important for parents to plan effectively.

Early intervention plays a key role in supporting children suffering from Autism. Research shows that identifying ASD early can pave the way for significant improvements, especially in communication. As a matter of fact, about two-thirds of preschool-aged children with autism show progress in language skills if early intervention is provided, especially when they receive the right kind of speech therapy. Physical therapy is also beneficial if started early, and it helps children develop motor skills like walking, coordination, and maintaining balance. Though early intervention services can be expensive, the long-term gains justify the investment.

Various therapies are available for individuals struggling with ASD, and each one tends to offer a different approach. For example, Applied Behavioral Analysis is widely used to encourage positive behaviors, promote social skills, and teach children how to apply what they've learned through their experience. On the other hand, occupational therapy (OT) helps children develop fine motor skills that are needed for daily activities like dressing, writing, or using utensils, and it also addresses sensory processing problems.

Then, there is speech therapy, which is led by licensed speech-language pathologists. This therapy is essential for improving communication in autistic individuals. It helps children express themselves and is most effective when integrated into the child's broader support system, which includes teachers, caregivers, and peers. Physical therapy focuses on improving gross motor skills and sensory integration, and it specifically targets challenges with movement, posture, and balance.

While each of these therapies offers a unique set of benefits that play a key role in a child's development, the associated costs can add up quickly. Understanding and anticipating such expenses is a crucial step in making informed decisions about your child's care. For a detailed look at the financial considerations for each therapy type, families must explore resources focused specifically on autism treatment costs.

Factors Affecting Therapy Cost

Understanding the factors that influence the cost of autism treatment can allow families to better prepare for the financial responsibilities that are involved in caring for a loved one with autism.

One key factor is the duration and intensity of therapy. Most therapies, including applied behavioral analysis, speech therapy, and occupational therapy, are billed on an hourly basis. The more hours a child requires each week, the higher the total cost will be. For example, ABA therapy typically costs anywhere between $120 and $150 per hour. Without insurance, this amount can add up to anywhere from $240 to $600 per day, or even $20,000 per month in some cases.[1]

On average, families of autistic children may end up spending up to $17,000 annually on behavioral interventions, with almost 25% of the families spending $30,000 or even more each year.

Another factor is the expertise of the therapist and the location where these services are provided. Therapists with specialized training oftentimes charge higher rates. Speech therapy, for example, can cost anywhere between $100 and $250 per hour, and occupational therapy may go from $100 to $200, depending on the therapist's experience, as well as the regional pricing differences.[2]

---

1. The cost of ABA therapy for autism. (n.d.). https://www.mastermindbehavior.com/post/cost-of-aba-therapy-for-autism
2. Autism therapy cost in new Jersey. (n.d.). https://www.mastermindbehavior.com/post/autism-therapy-cost

Location also plays a big role in determining the cost of treatment. Services in some of the big cities or high-cost areas tend to be more expensive than those offered in rural communities. Apart from therapy, the total cost of autism care may include healthcare, support services, and educational resources, and all of these costs can vary widely across countries and regions.

When planning for autism treatment, it's essential for families to take all of these factors into account so they may find effective and affordable care that meets their child's needs.

Cost Breakdown

When talking about the average cost of autism treatment, families often tend to consider several core therapies. The most common therapies in this regard are Applied Behavioral Analysis (ABA), Speech Therapy, and Occupational Therapy. Each of these treatments comes with its own unique pricing and factors that influence the cost of treatment.

Applied Behavioral Analysis (ABA)

Applied Behavioral Analysis is one of the most common therapies for children with autism. Its cost can vary greatly, but the average annual expense is somewhere between $40,000 and $60,000. Many families tend to spend about $17,000 a year on behavioral interventions, and roughly a quarter of those people tend to spend $30,000 or more. On an hourly basis, ABA usually costs somewhere between $120 and $150. Without insurance, daily costs can reach up to $600, while weekly totals can go up to $4,800, and monthly expenses can go beyond $20,000.

Speech Therapy

Speech Therapy is another important option in autism treatment. The cost of a single session can range from $100 to $250. However, it all depends on the therapist's expertise and location. Early and consistent speech therapy can pave the way for significant improvements. According to studies, two out of three preschoolers with ASD tend to improve their communication skills with early treatment.

Occupational Therapy

Occupational Therapy allows an individual with autism to develop motor skills, while helping them with everyday tasks. The average cost falls anywhere between $100 and $200 on an hourly basis, with rates depending on location, session duration, and the therapist's qualifications. These services may be available through schools, private providers, or even some of the early intervention programs. Some families may qualify for coverage through private insurance or Medicaid. [3]

---

3. Autism intervention costs. (n.d.). https://www.mastermindbehavior.com/post/autism-intervention-costs

Additional Treatment

While therapy makes up a large part of autism treatment costs, families should also consider the extra expenses that come with therapy. These expenses may include dietary interventions and educational support, which can significantly add to the overall financial burden of the child's family.

Dietary Interventions

Dietary interventions can range from minor dietary changes to more specialized and structured plans. Costs can go from $50 to $2,000 on a monthly basis, excluding the price of food. Managing all of these expenses requires careful planning and guidance from a professional healthcare provider or a nutritionist to make sure the chosen diet is safe and effective at the same time.

Educational Support

Educational support is another crucial but costly part of autism treatment. This may include special education programs, private tutoring, and therapy sessions. According to Total Care ABA, families may face additional medical costs ranging from $4,110 to $6,200 per annum. Some educational interventions, such as the Preschool Autism Communication Trial, can lead to long-term savings. While this may be more expensive initially, it can reduce unpaid care needs over time, thus easing the financial strain.[4]

Financial Assistance Options

Understanding the average cost of autism treatment can be challenging. However, there are several financial assistance options and resources that can help reduce the burden.

One viable option is the Medicaid Waiver Programs, also known as 1915(c) Home and Community-Based Services. Such programs tend to cover essential services such as medical treatments, transportation, in-home care, as well as respite services. They are designed specially to support individuals with autism living more independently.

Another program is the Supplemental Security Income (SSI). This program provides up to $791 per month for eligible children. Most states also offer Medicaid benefits for eligible children. Eligibility is based on factors like the severity of the child's condition and the family's income. For instance, a single-parent household must earn under $3,301 monthly, while a two-parent household must stay below $4,095 in order to qualify.

Tax deductions and credits can also assist families in managing autism-related expenses. Medical costs that go beyond 7.5% of a household's gross income may be deducted from federal taxes. This may include therapy

4. Kesherim, R. (2025, March 5). Is Autism Covered by Health Insurance: Benefits & Coverage. https://www.totalcareaba.com/autism/is-autism-covered-by-health-insurance

costs, doctor visits, medications, and even commuting. Furthermore, the Child and Dependent Care Credit provides up to $3,000 per dependent, or $6,000 in total for families that pay for child care while working or searching for work. This credit covers services such as after-school care and day camps.[5]

There are also several community grants and support programs available for families paying for autism treatment. The United Healthcare Children's Foundation (UHCCF) offers grants for families whose commercial insurance doesn't cover medical expenses. These grants can help pay for autism therapies, as well as the necessary equipment.

The MyGOAL Autism Grant Program provides yearly grants for U.S. families with children under 18 who suffer from autism. These grants can be used for therapy, educational support, or enrichment programs that aren't necessarily covered by insurance or schools, thus helping to bridge funding gaps.[6]

529A accounts, which are also called ABLE accounts, were created under the Achieving a Better Life Experience (ABLE) Act. These state-sponsored accounts help families save up to $15,000 per annum for long-term disability-related expenses without losing their eligibility for

---

5. What is the Child and Dependent Care Tax Credit? (2025, January 31). Fidelity. https://www.fidelity.com/learning-center/smart-money/child-and-dependent-care-tax-credit#:~:text=If%20you%20have%201%20qualifying,how%20many%20dependents%20you%20have.

6. MyGOAL Autism Grant program. (n.d.). MyGOAL. https://mygoalinc.org/mygoal-autism-grant-program/

government benefits such as Medicaid or SSI. While not federally tax-deductible, some states tend to offer tax breaks for contributions.

Together, these financial tools, governmental programs, tax benefits, grants, and savings accounts can significantly minimize the out-of-pocket costs of autism treatment. With the right kind of planning and support, families can easily manage the financial side of caring for a person with autism.

Final Word

The economic impact of autism treatment is significant. However, with early planning and awareness of available resources, families can find it easier to navigate the financial challenges. From therapy costs to additional care needs, and from public assistance programs to community grants, there are various options that can help ease such a burden. Empowering families with knowledge and support is key to ensuring that each and every child with autism has the opportunity to live a healthy life.

CHAPTER 14

BARRIERS TO CHANGE IN MEDICAL PRACTICE

Modern medical education, although comprehensive in so many ways, often falls short, especially when it comes to incorporating environmental determinants of health into its curriculum. If we look at it historically, we will realize that the focus has always remained on the biological and clinical aspects of disease. This includes things such as pathology, diagnostics, a nd pharmacological treatments. As a result, it leaves little to no room for exploring how environmental exposures, socioeconomic conditions, and climate change can impact human health.

If we look at this situation in a more systematic fashion, we will be able to identify three constant barriers to teaching public health and environmental health in undergraduate medical programs. These barriers include overcrowded curriculum, a lack of consensus and debate on what constitutes essential content, as well as insufficient institutional support.

Do you know what these barriers allude to? The truth is

that these issues reflect a broader systemic resistance to change within medical academia. While change is the only constant, with medical education, changes don't necessarily happen at a fast pace. As a result, the curriculum remains stale, and new research doesn't occur as much as it should. Well, that is just one of the many issues.

Another common issue with modern medical academics is that many curricula are designed with a disease-centric approach, which is fine, but more needs to be done. As a result, it fails to acknowledge the fact that prevention often begins with understanding the patient's environment, which ranges from air and water quality to housing conditions, as well as occupational hazards.

Along with these challenges, there also exists a widespread shortage of faculty that is trained in environmental health literacy. Without the right instructors who are equipped to teach this interdisciplinary subject, medical schools tend to struggle when it comes to delivering effective education in this domain. This educational gap leads to a generation of healthcare providers who may be less than prepared to recognize or address environmental contributors to illness. Whether it's lead exposure in children or heat-related illnesses in the elderly, there remains a persistent gap between what is and what should be.

Influence of the Pharmaceutical Industry on Research and Treatment

It is a well-known fact that the pharmaceutical industry enjoys a considerable influence over medical research, clinical guidelines, and therapeutic decisions. From 1999, all the way till 2018, pharmaceutical companies spent around $4.7 billion on lobbying the U.S. federal government, averaging $233 million on an annual basis. This financial power gives the industry a prominent voice in shaping healthcare policy, as well as funding priorities. [1]

This influence often results in a skewed focus toward high-revenue pharmacological treatments, sidelining research into prevention strategies or the environmental causes of disease. For instance, the development and promotion of drugs like Eli Lilly's orforglipron for weight loss illustrate a grand pattern. Industry investment often prioritizes treating the symptoms of chronic conditions rather than addressing their root causes. These causes can sometimes be industrial, and at other times, they relate to the lifestyles of individuals.

Moreover, pharmaceutical sponsorship of medical conferences, research studies, and even continuing medical education courses can cause conflicts of interest that subtly tend to guide clinical practices. Physicians may be more familiar with pharmaceutical solutions than with upstream

---

1. Wouters, O. J. (2020). Lobbying expenditures and campaign contributions by the pharmaceutical and health product industry in the United States, 1999-2018. JAMA Internal Medicine, 180(5), 688. https://doi.org/10.1001/jamainternmed.2020.0146

determinants of health like food deserts, toxic exposures, or less-than-adequate housing facilities. This dynamic gives birth to a reactive healthcare model rather than a proactive or preventive one.

Challenges in Implementing Prevention-Based Approaches

Transitioning from a treatment-centered to a prevention-oriented healthcare system presents a variety of structural and cultural challenges. In spite of growing evidence supporting the efficacy of preventive medicine, it is often overlooked and doesn't receive the right emphasis in both training and practice.

Overcrowded Curricula

The sheer amount of material medical students must master leaves little room for prevention or environmental health. Even when such topics are included, they often appear as electives or isolated modules rather than integral components of the core curriculum. It is very important for universities, the concerned authorities, and the relevant shareholders to understand the significance of such courses. They must use their influence to put rules in place that emphasize the importance of courses on environmental health and prevention.

Lack of Faculty Expertise

This is a sad state of affairs, but it is the hard truth. The people responsible for imparting information to future experts don't possess the right kind of capabilities. Without instructors who are well-versed in public health or environmental sciences, these subjects tend to be taught superficially or not at all. This lack of expertise paves the way for a cyclical problem. The educators who are responsible for sharing knowledge can't teach what they haven't been trained in, and new graduates aren't equipped with the right skills and resources to address environmental factors in their clinical work. Collectively, this creates a very hopeless situation not only for the medical academia but also for the health and well-being of the common folk who look up to doctors and health professionals for their assistance and support.

Institutional Resistance

It is time for institutions to let go of age-old teaching methods and pedagogies and to seriously consider modern health problems and their solutions. Many medical institutions remain entrenched in traditional models of education and healthcare delivery. As time passes, health issues evolve, and so must our approaches to addressing them. Relying on hackneyed research just won't cut it. Research funding, prestige, and clinical productivity often depend on specialization and high-tech interventions, not on prevention's slower, less-than-tangible outcomes. It is a matter of letting go of the old and embracing the new. This institutional conundrum can compromise the efforts that are needed to prioritize more holistic approaches to health.

Reimbursement Systems

While there are some great problems with the current medical system, one of the biggest problems is the poor reimbursement system. Current healthcare reimbursement models often tend to incentivize procedures and pharmacological interventions over things like counseling, prevention, or environmental assessments, which is not only harmful to the patients, but also brings down the overall level of the entire medical and academic fraternities. This economic disincentive discourages physicians from investing time in preventive care. As a result, they are more interested in treatment and medication, rather than addressing the root cause of the problems at hand.

Strategies for Integrating Environmental Factors into Medical Education and Practice

Despite these challenges, there are also some promising strategies that can facilitate the integration of environmental health into medical education, as well as practice:

Curriculum Redesign

Medical schools should spend time and resources on

integrating environmental health topics into existing courses, including pediatrics, internal medicine, and community health. Rather than treating them as add-ons or electives, such courses should be part of the compulsory courses. For instance, lessons on respiratory illnesses can include discussions of air pollution, while dermatology modules can explore the health impacts of climate change and exposure to UV rays.

Faculty Development

Investing in faculty training programs, workshops, and interdisciplinary collaborations can considerably improve the standard of environmental health education. Moreover, partnerships with schools of public health or environmental science departments can be particularly effective in building this capacity and helping it evolve into an established faculty.

Institutional Support

Like any other endeavor, teaching environmental factors in medical schools can be much more effective when there is institutional support. Leadership buy-in for long-term change is a must in some cases. Medical schools and teaching hospitals must allocate resources, both financial and logistical, in order to support curriculum innovation, faculty recruitment, and interdepartmental collaboration, which is extremely important in today's competitive world. Accreditation bodies can also play a powerful role by requiring competency in environmental health literacy.

Policy Advocacy

Health professionals can play a key role in advocating for educational reforms at the national and institutional levels. Organizations like the Association of American Medical Colleges and the National Environmental Education Foundation can serve as supportive allies in promoting systemic change in this area. In addition, aligning medical education with sustainable development goals and climate action frameworks can strengthen the case for integrating environmental content into training.

Community-Based Learning

Encouraging students and younger professionals to engage in community health projects focused on environmental justice or sustainability helps develop a real-world understanding of these issues. This experiential learning improves competencies and cultivates a sense of social responsibility among people who will be the opinion leaders and experts of tomorrow.

Final Word

Addressing the barriers to change in medical practice, especially the ones related to environmental health, requires a coordinated, multifaceted approach. Medical education needs to evolve beyond a biomedical model to one that embraces the entire spectrum of determinants that influence health.

Through curriculum reform, faculty development, institutional support, and advocacy, future physicians can be prepared to address the growing burden of environmentally-linked diseases and the responsibilities that come with them. Only by the integration of these dimensions into education and practice can the healthcare system become truly preventive, equitable, and responsive to the growing challenges of the modern-day era.

CHAPTER 15

POLICY REFORM FOR PREVENTION

It is a well-known fact that indoor air quality affects the health, comfort level, and productivity of building occupants. With time, building codes and standards have evolved to address issues related to ventilation, pollutant exposure, and energy efficiency. As scientific knowledge continues to grow and environmental goals shift, such regulations continue to change, and as they do, they influence the way HVAC systems are designed and installed.

In the early 1900s, concerns were raised about the spread of airborne illnesses, which resulted in the introduction of basic ventilation requirements. Early building codes would promote natural ventilation through some key features, like operable windows and taller ceilings. However, as time went by and as cities expanded and buildings became more sealed, mechanical ventilation systems became essential for maintaining indoor air quality.

While these systems were not as effective as natural ventilation, they served their purpose.

During the 1970s, energy shortages became more common, and this new shift prompted efforts to make buildings more energy-efficient by tightening their envelopes. While this improved energy conservation, it also played a key role in minimizing ventilation, further contributing to issues like sick building syndrome and a considerable increase in indoor pollutants. In the wake of these challenges, the need for regulations that balance energy savings with adequate ventilation has become heightened. This further led to the creation of ASHRAE Standard 62 in 1970 in order to define minimum ventilation requirements.

With time, the IAQ guidelines gradually broadened so they could address not just ventilation but also air filtration and pollutant control. Measures like the adoption of HEPA filters and MERV ratings improved the ability to filter out airborne particles. Organizations such as the EPA and OSHA started to set limits on workplace exposure to hazardous chemicals and particulates, thus enhancing the overall air quality standards.

The IAQ standards that we have today are closely linked to sustainability goals, with certifications like LEED and WELL, which promote the use of low-emitting materials, advanced filtration, and real-time monitoring. Standards like the International Mechanical Code and ASHRAE 62.1 are regularly updated in order for them to reflect current research on ventilation and energy-efficient HVAC technology.

As IAQ regulations continue to evolve, HVAC professionals need to stay in tune with the latest trends, thus ensuring compliance. This includes implementing demand-controlled ventilation, choosing high-efficiency filters, and performing regular system maintenance to maintain indoor air quality.

Policy Changes for Addressing Ventilation Issues

The U.S. Environmental Protection Agency has come up with some revised guidance on improving indoor air quality to limit the transmission of common respiratory viruses inside living spaces, schools, workplaces, as well as other indoor environments. These updates incorporate some of the latest scientific findings, and they align perfectly with recent ventilation recommendations from the Centers for Disease Control and Prevention.

According to Joseph Goffman, Assistant Administrator for EPA's Office of Air and Radiation, these revised guidelines will serve as a key resource for minimizing the spread of respiratory diseases within sealed spaces. He believes that improving indoor air quality is extremely important in protecting health alongside vaccinations, hand hygiene, and other preventive actions.

The updated recommendations offer a comprehensive approach to virus prevention, emphasizing improved ventilation through measures like opening windows and doors. The guidance also suggests upgrading HVAC filters, using portable air purifiers, and running fans to enhance air circulation, while using exhaust fans or attic fans to reduce airborne virus concentration. In addition, the EPA advises incorporating air treatment technologies, administrative policies, and regular cleaning and disinfection.

Understanding Indoor Air Quality and Its Impact

While many people are completely aware of the horrors of outdoor air pollution, indoor air pollution poses great health risks as well. Indoor air quality refers to the condition of the air inside buildings, directly affecting the comfort and well-being of occupants. Poor air quality can impact everyone, especially the vulnerable members of the population, like children, seniors, and individuals suffering from respiratory or cardiac conditions.

Managing indoor pollutants can significantly reduce health risks. Health effects may appear soon after exposure, or they may manifest themselves years later. The contaminants typically come from indoor sources that either emit gases or release particles, and insufficient ventilation can elevate the problem even further by failing to bring in enough fresh air or remove contaminants in an effective manner.

Respiratory viruses such as influenza, RSV, and the virus responsible for COVID-19 spread easily indoors due to the higher concentration of viral particles and close proximity between the occupants. These viruses lead to countless infections, which further results in hospitalizations and deaths.

Adequate ventilation and air filtration are two of the key elements in a multi-pronged defense against the spread of airborne viruses inside indoor spaces. Enhancing the flow of outdoor air into indoor spaces is an effective strategy to handle the problem of pollutants. When increasing ventilation isn't possible, using filters in HVAC systems or air cleaners can help minimize the number of airborne particles. It is essential to understand that no single IAQ method is sufficient on its own. Therefore, these strategies should be used together, alongside CDC-recommended health precautions, for your efforts to be most effective.

Role of Stakeholders

When it comes to putting together a policy for ventilation and indoor air quality, there are a few stakeholders that just cannot be ignored. Let's look at all the concerned parties in policy-making.

Government Agencies

Organizations such as EPA, CDC, WHO, and other local health departments play a crucial role in shaping IAQ and ventilation policies. These bodies are responsible for establishing national and regional standards. They also issue official guidance and enforce regulations via inspections and compliance checks. They also fund research initiatives and lead public health responses during times of crisis like pandemics, when effective indoor air management becomes critical.

Public Health Professionals and Experts

These individuals bring some of the most valuable evidence-based insights to the table. Their research and findings help identify the links between poor ventilation and respiratory problems, thus influencing important policy priorities. These experts and professionals also provide guidance on key ventilation parameters, such as recommended air exchange rates, in order to decrease the spread of airborne diseases, while improving public health outcomes.

Engineers, Architects, and HVAC Professionals

These professionals are essential in transforming IAQ policy into real-world applications. They are responsible for designing and installing building systems that support the right kind of ventilation, while incorporating energy-efficient solutions and advanced filtration technologies. These professionals assess the feasibility of brand-new IAQ measures and make sure that these structures comply with evolving technical standards.

Building Owners

These individuals are on the front lines of policy implementation. They are responsible for the maintenance of ventilation systems, and they also ensure ongoing compliance with health and safety regulations. Through stakeholder consultations, they offer practical input on operational challenges, as well as long-term maintenance needs, making them key partners in ensuring the effectiveness of IAQ improvements.

Educational Institutions

They have a duty to create safe and healthy spaces for students and staff. They work closely with government agencies to assess and upgrade school ventilation systems, and they often advocate for extra funding to modernize infrastructure. By involving teachers, parents, and community members, these institutions help increase awareness of the importance of IAQ inside school buildings and other educational institutions.

Labor Unions

Labor unions and employee advocacy groups tend to focus on ensuring safe working conditions, which includes air quality in indoor workplaces. They are responsible for advocating for enforceable IAQ standards in occupational health policies, while raising concerns when ventilation systems fail to deliver. Such groups often push for reforms that minimize health risks, as well as absenteeism, which is a product of poor air conditions.

Environmental and Community Advocacy Groups

These groups bring attention to the implications of

indoor air quality on the public, as well as environmental health. They work tirelessly to include IAQ in environmental justice conversations, while ensuring the marginalized communities are represented in their consultations. These organizations often monitor the impacts of development projects, while promoting sustainable building practices that are aimed at enhancing ventilation.

Academic and Research Institutions

Such institutions play a vital part in offering the scientific foundation for policy development. Through studies and findings on pollutant exposure, air quality trends, and health outcomes, these bodies supply important pieces of data that inform regulatory decisions. They also model potential policy impacts and offer independent, objective analyses to guide effective policymaking.

Industry Associations

Bodies like ASHRAE and REHVA set technical standards and also provide training for professionals who work in ventilation and IAQ-related fields. They play a crucial role in updating best practices, developing compliance guidelines, and also serving as a bridge between policymakers, professionals, and the general public.

General Public and Building Occupants

They are the most vital stakeholders whose lived experiences provide them with firsthand insight into the efficacy of IAQ measures. Through participation in consultations, community meetings, and regular feedback channels, they can advocate for improved air quality in homes, schools, as well as workplaces, thus ensuring that policies address real-world needs and concerns.

Final Word

The journey toward improved indoor air quality and ventilation policies is a comprehensive effort that requires intelligent policymaking, technological innovation, and active engagement of the stakeholders. As scientific understanding grows and environmental priorities evolve, the frameworks that govern how air quality is managed within our indoor spaces should also evolve.

From early ventilation standards to modern guidelines that integrate health, efficiency, and sustainability, the importance of clean indoor air has never been emphasized in such a way, especially in the wake of global health crises. It is important to understand that effective policies are not created in isolation. Instead, they depend on collaboration between government agencies, health experts, engineers, building owners, educational institutions, advocacy bodies, and the general public.

Each party plays a key role in shaping practical standards that protect public health and enhance overall well-being. As we move forward, the commitment to advancing ventilation systems and strengthening IAQ guidelines must be a shared priority across all sectors of society.

CHAPTER 16

FUTURE SCENARIOS AND IMPLICATIONS

Over the passage of decades, autism has actually become a prominent public health problem, with its prevalence rising globally. In the U.S., the prevalence of ASD among 8-year-olds increased from 0.66% in 2000 to 3.2% in 2022. This surge is attributed to a combination of broader diagnostic criteria, improved awareness, and enhanced screening practices.[1]

As we continue to look ahead, we can see that the trajectory of ASD prevalence is influenced by several factors, which include healthcare interventions, educational strategies, as well as environmental changes. In the upcoming sections, we will delve into projections of autism rates based on current trends and potential interventions. We will explore some key societal challenges that arise

---

1. Data and statistics on autism spectrum disorder. (2025, April 15). Autism Spectrum Disorder (ASD). https://www.cdc.gov/autism/data-research/index.html

from the increasing autism rates. Moving forward, we will also examine how climate change and continued modernization might impact such trends.

Projections of Autism Rates: Current Trends and Potential Interventions

Before moving toward interventions, let's examine some recent and current trends, along with also some projected scenarios. If we look at some of the more recent studies, we will realize that the new research indicates a significant rise in the prevalence of autism. Between the years 1990 and 2019, the global mean incidence of ASD in children under 5 years old was somewhere around 96.9 per 100,000, with the number slightly higher in males compared to females. In America, the prevalence among 8-year-old kids reached 3.2% in 2022, which was a considerable increase from 0.66% in the year 2000.[2]

Projections of ASD prevalence tend to vary. This fluctuation depends on several factors, which include diagnostic practices, societal awareness, and environmental influences. In a study focusing on the impacts of global warming on autism numbers from 1990 to 2019, it was found that a 1°C increase in temperature variation was directly associated with a 3% increase in the risk of ASD

---

2. Yang, L., Chen, F., He, X., Tong, Y., Li, Q., Yang, T., Peng, R., Wang, H., & Shi, Z. (2023). Global burden and inequality of autism spectrum disorders: Based on data from the 2019 Global Burden of Disease study. Preventive Medicine Reports, 36, 102511. https://doi.org/10.1016/j.pmedr.2023.102511

incidence. If you look at the Shared Socioeconomic Pathway (SSP) 585 scenario, which looks at high greenhouse gas emissions, the incidence of ASD is projected to increase significantly by 2100, especially in areas that have a latitude between 10° and 20°.

On the flipside, under the SSP126 scenario, which represents a pathway with low greenhouse gas emissions and sustainable development, the increase in ASD incidence is expected to be a little less pronounçed. According to this scenario, the projections indicate a less than 10% increase across all latitudes by the year 2100.

Impact of Interventions

The implementation of effective interventions can alter the trajectory of ASD prevalence. Early diagnosis and intervention are extremely important in improving developmental outcomes for individuals suffering from autism. According to research, early behavioral interventions can pave the way for improvements in communication, social skills, as well as adaptive behaviors. Furthermore, public health campaigns that are aimed at increasing awareness and decreasing stigma can encourage more individuals to seek diagnosis and support, which can potentially lead to improved outcomes and integration into the society that we live in.[3]

---

3. Fuller, E. A., & Kaiser, A. P. (2019). The Effects of Early Intervention on Social Communication Outcomes for Children with Autism Spectrum Disorder: A Meta-analysis. Journal of Autism and Developmental

Let's look closely at early behavioral interventions, especially the ones that are based on Applied Behavior Analysis. We will realize how these interventions led to substantial benefits in improving various aspects of development for children suffering from ASD.

Intellectual and Cognitive Improvements

A meta-analysis of 29 studies revealed that ABA interventions are highly effective in improving a person's intellectual abilities, with a visible improvement in IQ scores. These interventions also contributed to moderate improvements in non-verbal IQ and adaptive behaviors, including socialization and daily living skills.

Language and Communication Skills

Intensive early interventions, like the Early Start Denver Model, have shown amazing success in improving a person's language abilities. A study with children aged 18 to 30 months showed that people who received ESDM exhibited an average increase of 18 IQ points and 18 points in receptive language skills.[4]

In addition, a long-term study highlighted how children

Disorders, 50(5), 1683–1700. https://doi.org/10.1007/s10803-019- 03927-z

4. Dawson, G., Rogers, S., Munson, J., Smith, M., Winter, J., Greenson, J., Donaldson, A., & Varley, J. (2009). Randomized, Controlled trial of an intervention for toddlers with autism: The Early Start Denver model. PEDIATRICS, 125(1), e17–e23. https://doi.org/10.1542/peds.2009-0958

who underwent early intensive behavioral intervention maintained considerable language improvements over time, with younger children showing improved outcomes.

Social and Adaptive Behavior Enhancements

Behavioral interventions are effective, especially when it comes to improving social skills and adaptive behaviors in children with ASD. For instance, Pivotal Response Training focuses on enhancing pivotal areas like motivation and self-management, which leads to improved social communication and reduced disruptive behavior.

Moreover, early interventions can lead to better integration into regular education settings, with children displaying improved peer relationships and, more importantly, social competence.

Long-Term Benefits and Cost-Effectiveness

Not only does early intervention improve developmental outcomes, but it also offers long-term advantages. Children who receive early behavioral interventions are highly likely to achieve independence and require less intensive support as they grow older. This paves the way for reduced lifetime care costs and a better quality of life for autistic individuals.

Public Health Campaigns: Raising Awareness and Reducing Stigma

Public health campaigns play a key role in altering the trajectory of ASD prevalence by increasing awareness and decreasing stigma while encouraging early diagnosis and intervention.

Early Diagnosis

Campaigns that educate the public about the signs of autism can contribute to earlier identification and diagnosis of the problem. Early diagnosis is crucial, as it leads to timely intervention, which is associated with better developmental outcomes in autistic children.

Reducing Stigma and Encouraging Support-Seeking

The stigma surrounding ASD can prevent families from seeking diagnosis and support for their kids with ASD. Public health campaigns promoting understanding and acceptance can minimize this stigma, thus encouraging more families to access necessary services.

Enhancing Community Support

Campaigns can also mobilize community resources, which leads to the development of support networks for families with kids affected by ASD. Such networks can offer emotional support and share resources, which provide advocacy for necessary services while improving outcomes for individuals with ASD.

Societal Challenges Arising from Increasing Autism Rates

Healthcare Impacts

The rising prevalence of ASD is a big challenge for healthcare systems around the world. Individuals with ASD often require a variety of services, such as diagnostic evaluations, therapeutic interventions, and ongoing medical care. However, there are many healthcare systems that are less equipped to meet these needs.

A study published highlights several barriers to healthcare access for autistic individuals, which include shortages of specialized services, higher costs, and a lack of physician awareness. Such barriers can result in delays in diagnosis and treatment, adversely affecting the health and well-being of individuals suffering from ASD.[5]

Educational Impacts

Educational systems also face difficulties when accommodating the increasing number of students suffering from ASD. The inclusion of students with ASD in regular

---

5. Malik-Soni, N., Shaker, A., Luck, H., Mullin, A. E., Wiley, R. E., Lewis, M. E. S., Fuentes, J., & Frazier, T. W. (2021). Tackling healthcare access barriers for individuals with autism from diagnosis to adulthood. Pediatric Research, 91(5), 1028–1035. https://doi.org/10.1038/s41390-021-01465-y

classrooms requires resources like trained staff and specialized teaching materials. Without the right amount of support, students with ASD may experience difficulties in academic achievement and social integration.

Furthermore, the absence of standardized curricula and training for educators on ASD can contribute to inconsistent educational experiences for students. Implementing inclusive education practices for autistic children requires systemic changes in the overall educational structure, from policy reforms and teacher training to the allocation of resources to ensure that students with ASD receive the right kind of support.

Climate Change, Modernization, and Autism Rates

Climate Change and ASD Incidence

According to research, there is a direct connection between climate change and autism. A study analyzing data from the year 1990 all the way till 2019 found that increased temperature variation was associated with an increased risk of ASD, especially in regions with low socioeconomic development. This association may also be due to environmental factors like exposure to pollutants and nutritional deficiencies during pregnancy, which can affect the brain development of the fetus.

Modernization and Environmental Factors

Modernization, which is characterized by urbanization,

industrialization, and some significant changes in lifestyle, can lead to environmental exposures that may influence the development of ASD in younger children. Factors like increased exposure to air pollution, diet changes, and reduced physical activity have been identified as some of the key contributors to the rising prevalence of ASD.

Furthermore, modernization often contributes to changes in family structures and caregiving practices that can impact the early development of children. For example, increased screen time and lessened social interactions may affect social, as well as communication skills, thus contributing to the development of ASD in children.

Final Word

The trajectory of autism prevalence in the future is directly influenced by a combination of factors, which include healthcare interventions, educational strategies, as well as environmental changes. While projections indicate an increase in ASD numbers, particularly under high greenhouse gas emissions and limited mitigation efforts, implementing the right kind of interventions can alter such a trajectory. Early diagnosis and intervention, along with systemic changes in healthcare and education, are extremely important in addressing the challenges posed by the rising prevalence of ASD.

Moreover, understanding the potential impacts of climate change and modernization on autism rates is important in developing comprehensive strategies for mitigating these effects. By adopting sustainable practices and promoting awareness, societies can effectively work toward decreasing the number of ASD cases while ensuring that autistic people receive the support they need to thrive.

CHAPTER 17

EVIDENCE-BASED SOLUTIONS

Autism, or as most people call it, ASD, is a complex neurodevelopmental condition that manifests itself in a number of different ways. Children suffering from ASD may showcase persistent difficulties in social communication, restricted and repetitive behavior patterns, or loss of interest in activities. The symptoms of ASD may vary for different individuals, thus making early detection and intervention strategies even more essential.

According to the Centers for Disease Control and Prevention, almost 1 in 36 children in the United States is diagnosed with some kind of ASD. However, with time, we have seen that similar prevalence rates are emerging globally, which highlights the universality of this developmental challenge and the critical need for effective as well as scalable interventions.

After decades of intensive research, experts have deduced how important timely intervention is and how it can significantly influence outcomes in autistic children.

The earlier the support process begins, the greater the chances of improving language, social skills, academic performance, and long-term adaptive functions.

In the upcoming sections, we will delve deep into some fascinating real-world strategies that have demonstrated success both at the individual household level and within larger communities. From behavioral therapies to environmental changes and some holistic family-centered models, the evidence presented in the following paragraphs will show the transformative power of informed, timely, and contextually appropriate interventions.

In this chapter, we will also look at resources investigating the role of environmental factors during early neurodevelopment. Through some quantifiable case studies, clinical trial data, and meta-analyses, this chapter will build a strong case for adopting evidence-based and multidisciplinary approaches aimed at the needs of children and families affected by ASD.

Case Studies of Successful Interventions

1. Home-Based Interventions

Benhaven Family Support Program (USA)

Benhaven is a Connecticut-based non-profit organization that has been offering services to individuals with autism and other developmental problems since the year 1967. One of its key initiatives includes the Individual and Family Support Division, which delivers personalized and in-home services. This model believes in the philosophy of empowerment and giving families the tools and confidence they need to nurture autonomy, social inclusion, as well as daily functioning in their children.

Some of the key components of Benhaven's services are as follows.

- Respite care weekends: These initiatives offer families essential relief while ensuring continued support for the child's needs.
- Targeted skill-building activities: These activities focus on communication, social interaction, as well as tasks of daily life.
- Emergency support: This includes providing urgent supplies or crisis management strategies.

Between 2015 and 2020, outcome data revealed that 82% of families involved in this program reported considerable improvements in their children's communication skills, while 76% reported to have observed a reduction in behavioral disruptions. Furthermore, parents expressed increased confidence in managing challenging behaviors, while promoting their children's development independently. All of these findings show how consistent, home-centered support can result in sustainable progress.[1]

Parent-Mediated Early Intervention (PMEI)

A randomized controlled trial was published in The

---

1. Individual and Family Support Program | Benhaven. (n.d.). https://www.benhaven.org/programs/individual-and-personal-support

Lancet Psychiatry (Green et al., 2015). In this trial, a novel approach to early autism risk mitigation was introduced. It empowered parents to act as therapeutic agents in their child's development. The study brought together 54 infants who were at high risk of autism. Over five months, parents received structured coaching using video feedback, which helped them identify and respond more effectively to their child's social cues.

- At the age of 3, children whose parents received PMEI showed a 30% decline in ASD symptoms compared to the rest of the children in the control group.
- Cognitive and adaptive functioning gains persisted into early childhood, which demonstrated the intervention's effectiveness, as well as its long-term benefits.
- This study illustrates that even in the absence of a professional diagnosis, early modifications to the caregiving environment can effectively alter the developmental trajectory of children suffering from ASD.[2]

---

2. Green, J., Charman, T., Pickles, A., Wan, M. W., Elsabbagh, M., Slonims, V., Taylor, C., McNally, J., Booth, R., Gliga, T., Jones, E. J. H., Harrop, C., Bedford, R., & Johnson, M. H. (2015). Parent-mediated intervention versus no intervention for infants at high risk of autism: a parallel, single-blind, randomised trial. The Lancet Psychiatry, 2(2), 133–140. https://doi.org/10.1016/s2215-0366(14)00091-1

2. Community-Based Programs

The Buddies Program (United Kingdom)

Introduced by a UK-based organization called Dimensions, the Buddies Program provides a rich example of how structured social engagement can benefit young people suffering from autism. The initiative is aimed at individuals between ages 5 and 25 and includes weekend camping trips, home support, as well as community-based social clubs. Some of the key elements of this program include principles of peer modeling, mentorship, and personalized planning, which are tailored to individual strengths and interests. In this program, the participants participated in outdoor learning and sensory play, team-building activities, and recreational exercises of inclusion and resilience.

An internal evaluation that took place in 2021 revealed that 89% of participants showed improved social interaction, while 74% of the participants reported minimized social anxiety. Parents also highlighted gains in independence levels of their children, as well as adaptability, especially in new or unpredictable environments, which is oftentimes a key challenge for children on the autism spectrum.[3]

Enabling Through the Horse (Namibia)

In Windhoek, Namibia, a therapy program called

3. Best Buddies International. (2022, May 3). United Kingdom - Best Buddies International. https://www.bestbuddies.org/uk/

Enabling Through the Horse, led by Susan de Meyer, provides a culturally and contextually tailored approach to helping children with developmental issues. The program uses mounted and unmounted activities to enhance motor coordination, body awareness, and therapeutic engagement. In this program, the children participate in horse grooming and feeding, which makes them more responsible and teaches them balance and coordination skills. There are also interactive sessions that improve their communication with other people and animals.

Post-intervention reports from the teachers have revealed that a little over 60% of children demonstrated improved focus, while 50% developed enhanced expressive language skills within six months of weekly participation in the program. This program speaks volumes about the therapeutic effectiveness of animal- assisted interventions, especially in regions where traditional therapy resources are scarce.

Research Supporting Environmental Modifications

1. Environmental Enrichment

Environmental enrichment includes the introduction of diverse sensory stimuli, which include factors like textures, sounds, scents, as well as visual elements that promote brain plasticity and behavioral engagement. A 2015 study by Woo et al. randomly assigned 48 children between ages 3 and 12 years with ASD into two groups. The first group received standard behavioral therapy, while the children in the other group received sensory enrichment activities.

- Six months into the exercise, 42% of the enriched group showcased considerable symptom reductions.
- After 12 months in the program, 21% of children in the enrichment group no longer met the diagnostic criteria for ASD, which was remarkable.

These outcomes offer compelling evidence that the developing brain, especially in early and middle childhood, can be positively shaped by multi-sensory experiences when applied consistently and with structure.

2. Wraparound Services

The Wraparound Process is a team-based, family-driven framework of care, which is specifically designed to address the needs of children with behavioral health challenges, including ASD. It involves collaboration among caregivers, educators, healthcare professionals, as well as community agencies. A review by Bruns et al. (2010) highlighted the effectiveness of this model. The findings were as follows.

- There was a staggering 28% reduction in psychiatric hospitalizations.
- The program also contributed to a 21% increase in school attendance.
- 92% caregiver satisfaction rate, with families

reporting that services matched their specific needs

Unlike traditional care models with rigid program structures, the wraparound approach builds a flexible support system that is based on the child's strengths, cultural context, and family dynamics.[4]

Quantitative Data on Intervention Effectiveness

1. Behavioral Interventions

A meta-analysis of 65 randomized controlled trials was published in Autism Research in 2023. It evaluated the efficacy of several evidence-based behavioral models. The findings are as follows.[5]

Early Start Denver Model (ESDM):

In this model, an average gain of 17 IQ points was noticed during a period of two years. Moreover, there were some noticeable improvements in language development, as well as social reciprocity.

---

4. Definition and history of wraparound. (2025, March 6). Continuing and Professional Education | Human Services. https://humanservices.ucdavis.edu/wraparound-services/california- wraparound-standards-toolkit/history

5. Asf, & Asf. (2023, December 27). 2023 Year end review - Autism Science Foundation. Autism Science Foundation - Supporting and sharing autism research to improve the real lives of real people. https://autismsciencefoundation.org/2023-year-end-review/

Pivotal Response Training (PRT):

This training showcased a staggering 40% improvement in spontaneous verbalizations. Also, it is affordable and adaptable for use at home as well as in inclusive classrooms.

TEACCH Program:

This program saw a 30% increase in daily living independence, particularly in non-verbal children. Furthermore, it focused on structured teaching and predictable routines.[6]

2. Parent-Mediated Interventions in Asia

A meta-analysis conducted by Zhang et al. in 2022 examined 17 different studies from mainland China, Hong Kong, and Taiwan. This analysis evaluated the impact of culturally adapted, parent-led therapies. The findings were as follows.[7]

- The analysis saw a 23% improvement in children's social responsiveness.
- 19% gain in adaptive behavior scores.

---

6. Aba, B. S. (2025, March 14). Harnessing the TEACCH method for autism success. Brighter Strides ABA. https://www.brighterstridesaba.com/blog/teacch-method-for-autism/
7. Litson, K., Zhang, F., & Feldon, D. (2022). Zhang et al. (2022) Social Predictors of Doctoral Student Mental Health and Well-Being. OSF. https://doi.org/10.17605/OSF.IO/P7VJE

- Significant reductions in parental stress levels, as measured by standardized tools.

These results reinforce the global relevance and scalability of parent-mediated approaches, especially when they are adapted to reflect cultural and familial norms.

Final Word

It is important to understand that the journey of a child with autism is not predetermined. However, through deliberate, evidence-based strategies rooted in early identification, behavioral support, and improved environmental experiences, it is possible to foster meaningful, measurable progress in the developmental outcomes. As the case studies illustrate, effective intervention is not just limited to clinical settings; it can be used within homes, schools, communities, and even outdoors or in other contexts, some of which are even assisted by animals.

Furthermore, the latest research into environmental influences, like the impact of indoor air quality and prenatal exposure to carbon dioxide, is beginning to reshape our understanding of the early contributors to neurodevelopmental problems in little children. While science is still evolving, such theories underscore the significance of adopting a more holistic and interdisciplinary approach to autism care.

Moving forward, investment in community resources, professional training, cross-sector collaboration, and culturally responsive practices will be needed to increase the success of these interventions globally. By listening carefully to the voices of families and embracing innovation grounded in evidence, the path ahead promises great equity, empowerment, and opportunity for children with ASD.

CHAPTER 18

CREATING CHANGE: A COMPREHENSIVE ACTION PLAN

Autism is a real problem, and the numbers and facts shared in this book allude to the rampant pace at which this problem is spreading on a global level. So, how can this problem be taken care of? Well, there is no direct answer to this age-old question. After all, ASD in itself is a multifaceted condition. There are so many aspects to this condition that it is almost impossible for us to circumnavigate them all. However, while it seems difficult, a holistic approach can help parents mitigate the effects of ASD in their children.

While some of us may look at it as just another condition suffered by children, it is important to understand that ASD impacts the way a child lives life, let alone enjoys it, or makes full use of their capabilities. The inability to talk and express themselves, as well as their inability to socialize and make connections, is hard on a child, and even though it affects them on a daily basis, most parents and family members remain oblivious. This book serves as a comprehensive guide that will help identify the early signs in children, while offering timely intervention to prevent the harmful effects this condition may have.

When we talk about a holistic approach to dealing with autism, we must be able to look at all the contributing factors that may push a child toward developing ASD. Moreover, we must also be aware of the ways we can prevent this condition from flaring up while choosing the correct measures to fight it.

The thing about ASD is that it starts earlier in life. While some of the reasons are biological and genetic in nature, the environment and the lifestyle offered to the child also play a key role in affecting the child's neurodevelopment. Speaking of environment and lifestyle, it is crucial for parents to factor in the housing conditions.

Gone are the days when children would get the chance to play in open, lush green fields with fresh air, natural elements, and the absence of dust and pollutants. As villages turned to towns and towns to cities, the number of facilities available to the human race surely grew exponentially. While this modernization seemed like another step on the road to progress, it took away from us our right to enjoy the gifts and blessings that Mother Nature has in store.

With time, the houses transformed into tightly packed apartment complexes, and the spaces that should have been reserved for rest and recreation were taken over by huge commercial buildings. While no one can deny the effectiveness of the modern standards of living, one cannot deny the downsides of living in a tightly sealed space, with little or no natural air to bless our lungs.

In a sealed indoor space, it becomes easy for contaminants, pollutants, and gases to thrive. When there is a lack of fresh air inside living spaces, it becomes inevitable for the occupants to rely on electronic appliances for heating, air-conditioning, and ventilation. The overt use of machines results in the production of harmful gases such as carbon dioxide. With a lack of ventilation, smoke from someone's cigarette or from the stove can easily accumulate inside the house, making it hard for the occupants to breathe, thus resulting in respiratory and also cardiovascular diseases, which can build up over time.

Then, if a pet lover happens to live in these spaces, the fur they shed is likely to float around the house. While that soft cotton-like material may seem potentially harmless, it really isn't. It can cause skin allergies, runny eyes, coughing, sneezing, shortness of breath, and nasal congestion.

Apart from smoke, CO2, and pet dander, the lack of ventilation in living spaces allows mold and mildew to thrive. When you smell something pungent and musty inside your house, you mustn't take it lightly, for it can affect your health, as well as that of your children. Mold and mildew can also cause more serious problems like croup, pneumonia, and bronchitis.

Does it mean that children are the only ones at the receiving end of this less-than-healthy lifestyle? Not at all. However, the problem is that children are still in their developmental stages, and their immune systems are weaker than those of their older family members. When their system is attacked by pollutants and contaminants, they are more likely to develop serious problems that may weaken their bodily functions, and neurodevelopment is no exception.

Prolonged exposure to indoor contaminants and the lack of fresh and clean air can compromise a child's bodily functions, and over time, all of these things may manifest themselves into what we know as autism, or ASD.

Another key aspect in this regard is the kind of diet that ends up in a child's gut. As they say, you are what you eat. Back in the day, and also today, in some traditional societies, kids not only have access to fresh air and clean water, but they also have access to pure and unadulterated diets that help them grow perfectly, while making full use of their bodily capabilities and strengths. A balanced diet consisting of vegetables, fruit, meat, and dairy products is important so the children may receive their fair share of nutrients that are vital in their physical and mental growth.

In the so-called developed world, we live according to the rules and norms imposed upon us by the corporations that exist for the sole purpose of running their businesses and minting money, even if it comes at the cost of their customers' health. The food we eat, the bottled water we drink, and the medications that we take are infested with some of the most harmful and toxic chemicals. When those chemicals are infused into our systems, they can create some serious problems, and these problems can be inherited by our children. Hence, there has been a rise of autism cases around the world.

Another major cause of children contracting autism at a young age can also be attributed to a poor lifestyle. People who act irresponsibly during their youth are likely to engage in some kind of substance abuse. While some might smoke, others might drink, and some would even go the extra mile to take drugs that can potentially kill a human being. Little do they know that the harmful effects of those substances may be endured by their unborn children after they open their eyes to this mortal world.

While we have looked at some of the most common reasons behind ASD cases, how do we s2olve these problems? Well, the fact of the matter is that there is no direct answer to this question. In order to come up with an effective solution to the problem, we will have to go back to the beginning of this chapter, where we talked about a holistic approach to dealing with ASD.

It is high time now, and with countless cases of ASD in all corners of the world, the time has come for our society to join forces and create a focused consortium to tackle this problem effectively.

Parents, teachers, health professionals, pharmaceutical experts, and construction experts need to come onto the same page if we are to rid the world of ASD, a problem that tends to threaten the future of our upcoming generations. What's truly promising is to see how so many NGOs and focused groups are taking up this initiative, and doing everything in their capacity to curb the problem of ASD, which takes childhood away from children, and keeps them from living life to the very fullest.

Parents must invest in creating living spaces that are

safe for the kids and also energy efficient as much as possible. Besides safety and energy efficiency, the newly built homes should have adequate doors and windows for all fresh air to enter, thus eliminating the pollutants, contaminants, smoke, and gases that threaten the health of their children. They must also invest in CO2 sensors and high-quality HVAC systems that prevent extra exposure to this harmful gas.

Plants in the living space can be quite beneficial. A few pots of aloe vera inside the house can suck in the harmful gases inside the living space, thus keeping it safe and healthy for the occupants and their children. Moreover, it is also important not to invest in paints, carpets, furniture, and other household items that may give off VOCs, which can cause allergic reactions while causing asthma, liver and kidney damage, reproductive problems, and cognitive impairments in children.

If you have done all of the above and still find your child having a hard time speaking, communicating, solving problems, or cultivating strong relationships with other people, it is important to intervene early. Apart from taking them to the doctor, which is extremely important, parents can also take their kids to private, nonprofit, and community-driven programs that are aimed at helping children with developmental issues. Some common exam2ples of such programs include Benhaven's Family Support Program (USA), the Buddies Program (United Kingdom), and Enabling Through the Horse (Namibia).

Luckily, with the increase in awareness, people all around the world are understanding the importance of early intervention. Regardless of where you live in the world, you will find like-minded people who are interested in putting an end to this epidemic of autism that continues to threaten the future of our children and those who will come after them. The purpose of this book is to make this world a better place to live, where each and every child has access to facilities that can aid them in their development.

Now, with the help of social media, it has become even easier for parents of autistic children and those who want to prevent it in their kids to come together on a singular platform. On their social channels, they have access to experts who specialize in the area of autism, as well as informative and well-researched content.

Moreover, by leveraging the power of social media platforms like Facebook, YouTube, and Instagram, parents can communicate with each other and share their problems and experiences while offering suggestions and solutions that are backed by experience.

Remember, it is a fact that dealing with autism isn't easy. After all, it is a multifaceted problem, but we need to make it a part of our everyday discussions so that we can do something about it at a collective level. While the challenge is too great, it isn't insurmountable.

Through efforts, commitment, honesty, sincerity, compassion, and open conversation, we can provide our kids with a life and a world where they can fully utilize their gifts without lagging behind the rest of the crowd.

APPENDIX

Chapter 1

Section Title	Content Description
Rise of Autism	Access to better research and better diagnostics has led to the rise of autism cases. Living conditions and lack of access to fresh air and ventilation are among the causes.
Autism Rates Around the World	Numbers show that over 67 million people worldwide are affected by autism.
Autism Rates Since the 1960s	Today, the number is 100 times higher than in the 1960s.
Reasons for the Rise in Autism Cases	Hereditary factors, prenatal and environmental factors, and efficient diagnosis.

References

- Autism Statistics & Facts: How many people have autism? (n.d.). https://www.thetreetop.com/statistics/autism-prevalence
- National Autistic Society & National Autistic Society. (n.d.). What is Autism? https://www.autism.org.uk/advice-and-guidance/what-is-autism#:~:text=Autism%20is%20a%20lifelong%20developmental,and%20children%20in%20the%20UK.

Chapter 2

Section Title	Content Description
Structural Variances	Some of the key areas include cortical growth, cerebellum, and hippocampus.
Neuroanatomical Aspects	Neuronal connectivity, amygdala size differences, and neocortex alterations.
Air Quality, Pollution, and Brain Development	In the environment, we can find certain particulate matter that is not yet regulated, but it still exists, affecting the brains of our young ones.

References

- Autism and brain development interconnection. (n.d.-b). https://www.mastermindbehavior.com/post/autism- and-the-brain-development#
- Air quality impacts early brain development. (2020, December 5). School of Veterinary Medicine. https://www.vetmed.ucdavis.edu/news/air-quality- impacts-early-brain-development

Chapter 3

Section Title	Content Description
Combustion reaction of CO2	$O2 + CH4 \rightarrow CO2 + H2O$
Day-to-Day Activities Leading to CO2 Accumulation	HVAC, cooking, fireplace, laundry, soil underneath the house.
Myth of Good Indoor Air Quality	Construction materials, new furniture, carpets, and linens, which release chemical fumes, and this process continues for several weeks and even months.

References

- Schwartz, L., Guais, A., Chaumet-Riffaud, P., Grévillot, G., Sasco, A. J., Molina, T. J., & Abolhassani, M. (2010).

Carbon dioxide is largely responsible for the acute inflammatory effects of tobacco smoke. Inhalation Toxicology, 22(7), 543–551. https://doi.org/10.3109/08958370903555909

- The Headteacher | Better leadership, smarter spending. (n.d.). The Headteacher. https://www.theheadteacher.com/new-for-schools/the-impact-of-co2-on-childrens-learning

Chapter 4

Section Title	Content Description
Natural Ventilation vs. Artificial Ventilation	When compared to modern HVAC systems, natural ventilation can offer 10-30% more energy savings.
Building Standards Affecting Air Quality	Hydrofluorocarbons, or HFCs, are used for air-conditioning and refrigeration purposes. These chemicals are up to 1,000 times more dangerous than CO2 itself and contribute significantly to global warming.

References

- Air quality in the built environment - World Green Building Council. (2022, August 17). World Green Building Council. https://worldgbc.org/healthy-equity-resilience/air-quality-in-the-built-environment/

Chapter 5

Section Title	Content Description
Nature vs. Nurture	The brain tends to adjust and adapt based on the environment it is surrounded with.
Cell Growth, Migration, and Connection Formation	Neurons tend to move from the inner surface of the tube to the outer surface. The neurons are guided by the radial glia, which acts as scaffolding.
Blood Flow Patterns and Autism Developmental Windows	Most children tend to develop rapidly, showcasing different skills that emerge during specific developmental windows that start from birth and go all the way to the age of fourteen.

References

- Children's Hospital Los Angeles. (n.d.). Children's Hospital Los Angeles. https://www.chla.org/blog/experts/research-and-breakthroughs/what-can-blood-flow-tell-us-about-autism
- Kelly, Y., Kelly, J., & Sacker, A. (2013). Time for bed: associations with cognitive performance in 7-year-old children: a longitudinal population-based study. Journal of Epidemiology & Community Health, 67(11), 926–931. https://doi.org/10.1136/jech-2012-202024

Chapter 6

Section Title	Content Description
High CO2 Conditions and Clot Formation	It is a fact that high CO2 levels or hypercapnia can impact blood clot formation, thus influencing the body's hemostatic process.
Compromised Blood Flow and Poor Neural Tissue Development	If blood flow is blocked for any reason, it may very well lead to an ischemic stroke. Such a stroke damages brain tissue, and in some cases, it can even be fatal.
Why Do Conventional Treatments Fail with Developmental Interruptions?	Specific challenges include trauma, which impacts emotional regulation and attachment. Then, there is also neglect, which leads to developmental delays and brainstem damage, which prevents insight, making traditional therapies less effective.

References

- Kiray, M., Sisman, A., Camsari, U., Evren, M., Dayi, A., Baykara, B., Aksu, I., Ates, M., & Uysal, N. (2014). Effects of carbon dioxide exposure on early brain development in rats. Biotechnic & Histochemistry, 89(5), 371–383. https://doi.org/10.3109/10520295.2013.872298

- Burch, G. E., & De Pasquale, N. P. (1965). The effect of CO2 on the viscosity of whole blood. Archiv Für Kreislaufforschung, 46(1–4), 161–167. https://doi.org/10.1007/bf02120179

Chapter 7

Section Title	Content Description
CO2 Accumulation in Traditional Cribs	Most cribs use padded bumpers. Such bumpers are usually made of multiple layers of fabric, often wrapped around fiberfill or other cushioned materials.
Safer Alternatives	Breathable Bumper, Minimalist Bedding, Mattresses with Ventilation Holes.
Improving Air Quality in Your Baby's Room	The first thing you can do is monitor indoor air quality using a device like the IQAir AirVisual Series.

Chapter 8

Section Title	Content Description
Requirements for Effective CO2 Removal	First of all, ventilation can be achieved by opening the windows and doors, as well as using an HVAC system.
Mathematical Models for Gas Behaviors and Airflow Patterns	These models often use partial differential equations. Such models can either be parabolic or hyperbolic.
Floor Level Ventilation	When the wood absorbs too much moisture, it tends to expand beyond its natural limits, thus causing the boards to bow or warp. Not only does this affect the visual appearance of your flooring, but it also compromises the structural integrity of the flooring.

References

- The Reynolds-Averaged Navier-Stokes (RANS) Equations and Models. (n.d.). System Analysis Blog | Cadence.
- https://resources.system-analysis.cadence.com/blog/msa2021-the-reynolds-averaged-navier-stokes-rans-equations-and-models
- Le2mon, M. (2025, February 3). CO2 safety in restaurants, bars, venues. CO2 Meter.
- https://www.co2meter.com/blogs/news/co2-safety-in-restaurants-bars- venus#:~:text=In%20general%2C%20the%20American%20Society%20of%20Heating%2C,CO2%20levels%20be%20maintained%20below%201%2C000%20ppm.

Chapter 9

Section Title	Content Description
Autism in Traditional Communities	Cleaner air, better ventilation, minimizing exposure to toxins, and lifestyle factors that differ from those in urbanized, industrialized areas.
Global Trends in Autism Diagnoses	Between the years 1990 and 2019, the global prevalence of autism increased by a staggering 39.3%.
Sleeping Practices, Infant Care, and Autism Rates	In regions and cultures where co-sleeping is common, such as Japan, India, and some major parts of East Asia, infants often share a bed or a room with their parents for an extended period until they reach a certain age.

References

- Davidovitch, M., Slobodin, O., Weisskopf, M. G., & Rotem, R. S. (2020). Age-Specific Time Trends in Incidence Rates of Autism Spectrum Disorder following adaptation of DSM-5 and Other ASD-Related Regulatory Changes in Israel. Autism Research, 13(11), 1893–1901. https://doi.org/10.1002/aur.2420

- Russell, G., Stapley, S., Newlove-Delgado, T., Salmon, A., White, R., Warren, F., Pearson, A., & Ford, T. (2021b). Time trends in autism diagnosis over 20 years: a UK population-based cohort study. Journal of Child Psychology and Psychiatry, 63(6), 674–682. https://doi.org/10.1111/jcpp.13505

Chapter 10

Section Title	**Content Description**
Autism in Traditional Communities	Cleaner air, better ventilation, minimizing exposure to toxins, and lifestyle factors that differ from those in urbanized, industrialized areas.
Global Trends in Autism Diagnoses	Between the years 1990 and 2019, the global prevalence of autism increased by a staggering 39.3%.
Sleeping Practices, Infant Care, and Autism Rates	In regions and cultures where co-sleeping is common, such as Japan, India, and some major parts of East Asia, infants often share a bed or a room with their parents for an extended period until they reach a certain age.

References

- Isaacs, N. P. (2024). 'The window area shall be at least one-tenth of the area of the room': The origins of a daylight (and ventilation) requirement in modern building codes. Lighting Research & Technology, 56(6), 637–659. https://doi.org/10.1177/14771535231225363 Russell, G., Stapley, S., Newlove-Delgado, T., Salmon, A., White, R., Warren, F.,

Pearson, A., & Ford, T. (2021b). Time trends in autism diagnosis over 20 years: a UK population-based cohort study. Journal of Child Psychology and Psychiatry, 63(6), 674–682. https://doi.org/10.1111/jcpp.13505

- TEN Key Daylight & Electric Light Metrics. (n.d.). https://www.iesve.com/discoveries/article/3813/ten-key-daylight-and-electric-metrics

Chapter 11

Section Title	Content Description
Infant Sleep Patterns and Brain Development.	Newborn babies tend to spend a significant chunk of their sleep in what we call the Rapid Eye Movement (REM) sleep, which is a crucial process for brain development.
CO2 Accumulation and Sleep Environments	CO2 is produced naturally when a human breathes, and it is expelled from the room through ventilation or air circulation.
The Impact of Sleep Environment on CO2 Levels.	In a traditional crib, especially when the crib is enclosed by a bumper or placed in a poorly ventilated room, CO2 buildup is highly likely to occur.

References

- News-Medical. (2020, April 21). Atmospheric CO2 levels can cause cognitive impairment. https://www.news-medical.net/news/20200421/Atmospheric-CO2-levels- can-cause-cognitive-impairment.aspx TEN Key Daylight & Electric Light Metrics. (n.d.). https://www.iesve.com/discoveries/article/3813/ten- key-daylight-and-electric-metrics
- Gutierrez, J. (2025, March 17). Managing ideal indoor humidity level to prevent mold growth | GP inspections. Guaranteed Property & Mold Inspection. https://www.gpinspect.com/article/humidity-level-to- prevent-mold/

Chapter 12

Section Title	Content Description
Prevention Strategies	Authorities like the Health and Safety Executive (HSE) and the Department for Education (DfE) recommend that all occupied areas in early years settings be properly ventilated, without compromising the comfort of learning and play environments.
Daily Routines and Practices	Ventilation, cleaning, indoor plants, air purification.
CO2 Monitoring	When choosing a device to monitor CO2 levels, you have two main options, i.e., dedicated CO2 monitors and air quality monitors.

References

- AQI Basics | AirNow.gov. (n.d.). https://www.airnow.gov/aqi/aqi- basics#:~:text=When%20AQI%20values%20are%20above,also%20has%20a%20specific%20color.
- Kane International. (n.d.). What are safe levels of CO and CO2 in rooms? | Kane International Limited. Kane International Limited. https://www.kane.co.uk/knowledge-centre/what-are-safe-levels-of-co-and-co2-in-rooms

Chapter 13

Section Title	Content Description
Factors Affecting Therapy Cost	The duration and intensity of therapy.
Cost Breakdown	The most common therapies in this regard are Applied Behavioral Analysis (ABA), Speech Therapy, and Occupational Therapy. Each of these treatments comes with its own unique pricing and factors that influence the cost of treatment.
Financial Assistance Options	There are also several community grants and support programs available for families paying for autism treatment. The United Healthcare Children's Foundation (UHCCF) offers grants for families whose commercial insurance doesn't cover medical areas.

References

- Autism intervention costs. (n.d.).
- https://www.mastermindbehavior.com/post/autism-intervention-costs
- Kesherim, R. (2025, March 5). Is Autism Covered by Health Insurance: Benefits & Coverage. https://www.totalcareaba.com/autism/is-autism- covered-by-health-insurance

Chapter 14

Section Title	Content Description
Influence of the Pharmaceutical Industry on Research and Treatment	From 1999, all the way till 2018, pharmaceutical companies spent something around $4.7 billion on lobbying the U.S. federal government, averaging $233 million on an annual basis.
Challenges in Implementing Prevention-Based Approaches	Overcrowded Curricula, Institutional Resistance, Reimbursement Systems.
Strategies for Integrating Environmental Factors into Medical Education and Practice	Institutional support, policy advocacy, and community-based learning.

References

- Wouters, O. J. (2020). Lobbying expenditures and campaign contributions by the pharmaceutical and health product industry in the United States, 1999-2018. JAMA Internal Medicine, 180(5), 688. https://doi.org/10.1001/jamainternmed.2020.0146

Chapter 15

Section Title	Content Description
Influence of the Pharmaceutical Industry on Research and Treatment	From 1999, all the way till 2018, pharmaceutical companies spent something around $4.7 billion on lobbying the U.S. federal government, averaging $233 million on an annual basis.
Challenges in Implementing Prevention-Based Approaches	Overcrowded Curricula, Institutional Resistance, Reimbursement Systems.
Strategies for Integrating Environmental Factors into Medical Education and Practice	Institutional support, policy advocacy, and community-based learning.

Chapter 16

Section Title	Content Description
Projections of Autism Rates	In America, the prevalence among 8-year-old kids reached 3.2% in 2022, which was a considerable increase from 0.66% in the year 2000.
Impact of Interventions	According to research, early behavioral interventions can pave the way for improvements in communication, social skills, as well as adaptive behaviors.
Raising Awareness and Reducing Stigma	Public health campaigns play a key role in altering the trajectory of ASD prevalence by increasing awareness and decreasing stigma, while encouraging early diagnosis, as well as intervention.

References

- Dawson, G., Rogers, S., Munson, J., Smith, M., Winter, J., Greenson, J., Donaldson, A., & Varley, J. (2009). Randomized, controlled trial of an intervention for toddlers with autism: The Early Start Denver model. PEDIATRICS, 125(1), e17–e23. https://doi.org/10.1542/peds.2009-0958

www.ingramcontent.com/pod-product-compliance
Lightning Source LLC
LaVergne TN
LVHW100306210926
848480LV00003B/1038